Miracle of an Ordinary Guy
STORIES OF A CANCER SURVIVOR

MICHAEL ALTENHOFF

Printed in the United States of America
First Printing, 2018

Production by: Nikki LoBue, Scholastica Nguyen and Jenny Williams

You can continue following my journey via my blog at
www.mikealtenhoff.com

Table of Contents

TO MY LOVING WIFE,

WHO NEVER ALLOWED ANYONE TO THINK

'GOODBYE' WAS AN OPTION.

FOREWORD

You have **CANCER**

These words caught your attention, right? Well, I want to share a message with each person affected by the news of my diagnosis and some words of inspiration to strangers whose lives changed in a moment as mine did.

"You have cancer." These three words are difficult to hear when the news involves a friend who requires your support. But when *you* have cancer, the most immediate response is "I will fight it! I will beat cancer." It is as though we have been conditioned to respond with this phrase. From the beginning, however, I questioned the popular response. I don't even remember having a reaction because everyone usually reacted for me with their version of "Kick cancer's butt," "You will beat this!" or "If anyone can do it, it's you. You are so strong." My oncologist tried assuring me the news was good news because my type of cancer was slow growing and highly curable.

I questioned the responses from the beginning because there was no opponent in the boxing ring waiting to spar with me, waiting to present its butt for me to *kick*. Cancer didn't have a face until I saw the tear run out of my eye while looking in the mirror. If a single tear can be filled with so much emotion, then how, I wondered, could I begin to fight the billions of cancer cells inside my own body. I didn't know what to do, so I did what I trained to do in the Army: complete the mission step by step.

This is my story. For the better part of 48 years, I have opened my heart and mind only to a select few. My life defines the word introvert. But now I hope to share my experiences through this book to make you smile, cry, laugh, question, and simply say "Wow, that is weird." Trust me, a few of the stories I share are just *out there*.

My goal in sharing these stories is to fulfill a promise from my family and friends to remember the memories this experience brought us. I begin my story with this poem by an unnamed author:

> I asked for Strength…
>
>> And God gave me Difficulties to make me strong.
>
> I asked for Wisdom…
>
>> And God gave me Problems to solve.
>
> I asked for Prosperity…
>
>> And God gave me a Brain and the ability to work.
>
> I asked for Courage…
>
>> And God gave me Danger to overcome.
>
> I asked for Love…
>
>> And God gave me Troubled people to help.
>
> I asked for Favors…
>
>> And God provided me Opportunities.
>
> I received nothing I wanted
>
>> But received everything I needed.

CHAPTER ONE

It's All in the Numbers

I never understood why I needed to take my socks off before surgery when the surgical area was all the way up in my armpit area. It didn't make sense to have to endure the added discomfort of cold feet. In fact, the entire surgery didn't make sense to me logically. The 20-minute procedure was to cut out a piece of fatty tissue that didn't cause any pain in the first place. But, back to the socks. I attempted to reason with the nurse with a reasonable argument: the socks protected me against hospital germs that could enter the pores of my feet and land me in a quarantine room within the Center for Disease Control suffering a disease not seen since the bubonic plague. The nurse was unconvinced and answered by commanding with the same energy as Moses' parting the Red Sea "Off with the socks!"

I climbed up on the gurney and watched the constant flow of medical staff pass in front of me. I was sure one of them would notice me lying there shivering with no socks and an open-back hospital gown flapping in the breeze of the air conditioner blowing down on me. No.

Finally, the anesthesiologist approached and began searching both hands looking for a suitable vein to start the IV. I couldn't resist suggesting that with socks on I'd be warmer, and he would then have his choice of a number of veins. Without so much as a grunt, he ignored me and poked the needle into my hand with all the tender kindness of a movie villain about to inject me with truth serum. I guess he knew what he was doing because he hit the vein on the first try. So, there I lay sockless and shivering all set and waiting for the surgeon to arrive.

Let me reflect for a moment because this story actually began six weeks earlier (good thing the Army trained me well to "hurry up and wait") in late August 2015. I had just completed my annual physical with my primary doctor with good news. My cholesterol levels were finally within the good range and my weight was down approximately 20 pounds since April. Before jumping off the table, I asked the doctor to take a quick look at a lump below my left armpit area.

I raised my left arm above my head as if I were reaching for a rung on a ladder. I used my right hand to grab the lump and explained that I had noticed it back in April but forgot to say anything about it. I didn't experience any pain from it and didn't think it grew at all but only became more noticeable due to the weight loss.

The doctor approached and grabbed the skin tissue, pushed it in circles and in and out. I reported no pain. We repeated the process of raising and lowering the arm followed by the prodding three or four times. He took his gloves off and started talking as he rinsed his hands. He diagnosed the lump as "lipoma." Lipoma is a benign tumor (not cancerous) most commonly found in adults 40–60 years of age. There is no known cause of a lipoma tumor, but I obviously didn't care for the description "fatty tissue." The doctor put me at ease by explaining that skinny people get lipoma tumors also — so HA!

I put my shirt on and was uttering the words "see you next year" when the doctor handed me the business card of a surgeon and said, "Go see this surgeon for a second opinion just to make sure."

Nothing is ever easy!

Three weeks later, after a full day at work and a race through congested traffic, I sat in a chair in the surgeon's exam room… waiting. It really does make it easier when the surgeon actually has bedside manners and takes an interest in you as a person. He came in and asked about what I did for a living and my family background and joked about what I had been doing the last 47 years of my life. He sat and genuinely listened. I was so comfortable with our conversation that I was about to leave before showing him the lump that brought me to the office. But no. I stripped off my work shirt and lifted both arms as he started to ask which arm it was.

"Never mind," he said, stopping and fixing his stare on my left arm. He stood up and walked directly to me and said, "Lipoma." I told him it didn't hurt but I could feel it while swinging my arms after losing some weight over the summer. The surgeon recommended the removal of the lipoma based on the fact that they never go away on their own. I agreed and that's how I ended up sockless and shivering waiting for him in the pre-surgery room.

Now, back to the present. The surgeon sat down and introduced himself to my wife, Diana, as Mark. He asked if I had any questions. I had no questions, but asked him to put Diana at ease by explaining that lipoma surgery is no big deal. The surgeon obliged, explaining how common lipoma is and the various locations they are found on the body. It is simply fatty tissue and *not* cancerous, he said, and there is a 1 in 1,000,000 chance the lipoma was anything else.

I looked at the clock: 10:40AM.

At 10:48AM I was freezing in the operating room without my socks on waiting for the doctor to arrive and reminding the anesthesiologist not to allow me to wake up halfway through surgery.

At 11:30AM I woke up in the recovery room, and when I turned my head to the right Diana said, "You have cancer!"

Yes, it happened that quick.

* *

The American Cancer Society estimates 1 in 2 males in the United States will develop an invasive site cancer.

* *

From that moment on cancer showed up at every turn of my head. On the drive home I heard radio commercials about cancer, saw billboards requesting support for cancer, and listened to news stories announcing medical breakthroughs for the war on cancer. Cancer was in my every thought as I waited for the "official" diagnosis.

The three days following surgery I was in a training class at work. During lunch on the third day the much-anticipated phone call came in from the surgeon.

Surgeon: "Hi, Mike, this is Mark. The lab work came back from the biopsies I took on Monday."

Me: "Before you tell me about the diagnosis, I have to tell you that you are fired from pre-game speeches. The whole *1-in-a-million* thing didn't quite work out."

Surgeon: "Yeah I would have to agree with you. I've been a surgeon for 33 years, and this surgery was a surprising find. I suspected something might be abnormal when you were going through pre-op procedures and we placed your arm above your head. The lump just didn't look the same as it did in the office. I made the incision and knew instantly that it was cancer."

Me: "How did you know?"

Surgeon: "The consistency of the lymph node area. It was yellowish and looked like popcorn."

Me: "Did the definitive results come back from the lab?"

Surgeon: "Well, the lab results came back as Hodgkin Lymphoma, but the pathologist couldn't get a positive result. We're forwarding the biopsies to The Cleveland Clinic where they have a specific dye for Hodgkin's classification."

The surgeon ended the call by giving me the name of an oncologist who came highly recommended.

· ·

**1 in 417 males in the United States
will develop Hodgkin Disease cancer.**

· ·

The lifetime risk of developing or dying from cancer refers to the chance a person has, over the course of his or her lifetime (from birth to death), of being diagnosed with or dying from cancer. These risk estimates, along with annual incidence and mortality data, are another measure of how widespread cancer is in the United States.

Here are the odds of my cancer numbers:

- † American Cancer Society classifies Hodgkin Lymphoma as RARE, accounting for only 0.5% of all new cancer cases in the US.

- † Hodgkin Lymphoma is further classified in four subgroups with a RARE 5.0% identified as nodular lymphocyte-predominant Hodgkin Lymphoma.

Although the prognosis is good with a 90–100% remission rate with primary therapy, relapse is common as some 10–15% of patients see a re-occurrence on average 3–6 years after diagnosis. The overall 10-year survival rates are >90% in limited stage disease.

CHAPTER TWO

Faith for My Fears

The treatment of my cancer turned out to be the greatest enemy to my health. On February 25, 2016, a chemotherapy drug called bleomycin that was intended to save my life nearly claimed it as my life functions began to shut down. Bleomycin inhibits DNA metabolism and is used as an antineoplastic — a drug that prevents the multiplication of cancer cells — especially for solid tumors. I managed to get every side effect in each band of risk starting with the most common ones that occur in >30% of patients:

- † Fever and chills

- † Skin reactions: redness, darkening of the skin, stretch marks on the skin

- † Nail thickening, nail banding

- † Hair loss

I also experienced these less-common side effects that occur in about 10–29% of patients:

- † Nausea and vomiting

- † Poor appetite and weight loss

✝ Mouth sores

✝ Lung problems: pneumonitis

And I was not spared the most rare side effects that occur in <10% of patients:

✝ Pulmonary fibrosis, which may cause severe or life-threatening lung problems

When I arrived at the appointment to receive chemotherapy infusion #10, for the first time the oncologist placed a pulse oxygen monitor on my finger and noted that my oxygen level was below 85%. He called the hospital and arranged to admit me for observation. I went home and packed some clothes and got ready to head to the hospital. I thought I felt okay, the real indication that I was not okay was that I asked to be dropped off at the door because I didn't think I could make the walk in from the parking lot. I sat down in the lobby and waited for my wife to join me at the registration table... and do not remember anything from that point on. Here's a quick summary of what others told me took place:

✝ I was admitted to a regular room for assessment, had trouble maintaining oxygen levels >85%, developed a fever of 106, and was submersed in ice baths and intubated.

✝ I then spent 6 weeks in the ICU as they attempted to diagnosis the cause of my life-threatening symptoms; during this time, I underwent surgery to insert an airway tracheotomy tube and a feeding tube.

✝ I was transferred to a specialty hospital for three-and-a-half months where I was weaned off the ventilator and began rehab for muscle atrophy and speech problems, including swallowing.

✝ I was transferred to an acute rehab hospital for five-and-a-half weeks where a lung-function test revealed the loss of nearly 80% of my lung capacity due to irreversible scarring (fibrosis).

✝ In August, some six months after I was scheduled for infusion #10, I finally came home in a wheelchair requiring 4L of oxygen with no movement and 8–10L of oxygen for standing, rolling the wheelchair, and eating. I required supplemental oxygen for *everything* you take a breath for.

Life had become a series of challenges. I could not live on my own because I was unable to be in an upright position for more than 90 seconds at a time. I did not drive because I had such severe neuropathy that I could not feel my right foot most of the day. I had developed anxiety from my experiences in the hospital and in the ICU and left my room only four times. To get an idea of what it was like, imagine yourself being confined to a locked box and feeling your chest burning for oxygen with every effort to move.

I had become a burden to those who loved me the most. Sure, I learned early to ask for help and believed that people responded because they wanted to help. We were blessed by so many families who offered their support by cooking meals, caring for the kids, and even driving out of their way to visit me. I tried to listen attentively to family members' moving around the house so I could time my 1,013th request for some help — handing me my toothbrush or a cup of water to wash down pills or emptying the urinal because I couldn't make it to the bathroom. They always did it with a smile, no matter how many times I asked, but it was tearing me apart.

In one of my darkest moments in the hospital, I lay in bed alone and crying. I broke down and texted these words:

> I'm in a bad mental state right now. Probably a good thing I have no mobility.

Followed by:

> I don't want this life anymore. I'm alone, uncomfortable and things weren't supposed to be like this.

I prayed every night, always beginning with the Lord's Prayer and thanking him for the wonderful support of my family and friends who made time for me. But I began to question whether I truly knew how to pray. I broke my regular approach and talked to God as a friend:

> Father, my heart is heavy. I feel like I have to carry the burden alone. My thoughts are occupied with an impending sense of doom. Words like "exhausted," "distraught," and "overwhelmed" seem to describe where I am. I am not sure how to let you carry my heavy load, so please show me how. Take it from me. Let me rest and be refreshed so my heart won't be so heavy in the morning.

My mind wandered from prayer to reflection on 2 Peter 3:8: "But, beloved, be not ignorant of this one thing, that one day

[is] with the Lord as a thousand years, and a thousand years as one day." I often chose to ignore this lesson during the recovery period. I attempted instead to bring God into my timeline by announcing discharge dates of Mother's Day, Memorial Day, and finally the annual family 4th of July barbecue. It was at that point that I realized I was losing the fight with my self-pity and spirit-destroying timelines.

I made the sign of the cross and then fell asleep.

When I woke up I seemed to have a clear understanding of my misdirected steps causing my anxiety. God is not a genie in a bottle. We cannot rub the lamp and get our wishes granted. You see, God is always loving — and His love is unconditional. If I remember His love, then I should also remember the following parable:

> There was a man who lived in a house next to a river.
>
> After a heavy storm, the water rose, and an announcement came over the radio urging locals to leave their houses before their homes were flooded.
>
> "Oh, no," said the man confidently to himself. "I am a religious man, I pray, God loves me, God will save me."
>
> The water rose higher, and the man was forced to move into the second story of his house. A fellow in a row boat came along and called for the man to hurry and get into the boat.
>
> "Oh, no, that won't be necessary," the man insisted. "I am a religious man, I pray, God loves me, God will save me."

Finally, the house was completely engulfed in water, and a helicopter swooped in to rescue the man, now perched on the roof.

Again he refused, saying, "I am a religious man, I pray, God loves me, God will save me."

Just then, a huge wave of water swept over the house, and the man drowned.

When he got to Heaven, he demanded an audience with God.

"Lord," he said, "I am a religious man, I pray. I thought you loved me. Why did this happen?'

"What do you mean?" the Heavenly Father asked. "I sent a radio announcement, a boat, and a helicopter, and you still wouldn't listen to me!"

Was I the man with the flooded house? Was I looking for God to speak to me through a burning bush or perform an instant miracle healing? Was I simply not paying attention?

To help you understand what happened next, I need to explain what my therapy sessions at the hospital were like. The scarring in my lungs restricts both of my lungs from expanding fully to allow me to get a deep breath, and the lung capacity is limited to holding 20% air volume. The best way I can explain how it feels is for you to imagine taking a belt and tying it around your chest and pulling it tight. Next, put on a swimmer's nose clamp to decrease the ability to take in air through your upper airway. Now, with the belt around your chest and the clamp on your nose, try to swallow some food, brush your teeth, or talk.

Difficult? Well, you're not done yet: Now try to *exercise*!

That said, the pain I experienced in performing therapy was probably more mental than physical. I would get so worked up with anxiety on Friday night anticipating therapy to come the following Monday. Therapy session times were posted on the room door on the date of exercise. I looked at my posted therapy time with dread — waiting for the torture to begin. The knock came, and two therapists would enter with the intention of getting me simply to sit at the edge of the bed with my feet on the floor, knees bent with thighs parallel to the floor and back straight up at 90 degrees. The goal was to build core muscles and retrain my breathing pattern. But here's how I interpreted the therapy:

> My hands are bound behind my back with the back of my wrists touching and secured with a thick black nylon zip cord. I fight with what little muscle I have as the torturers attempt to lift me to the upright sitting position. I thrash about in their grip and attempt to plea that I'm not ready or that I need my music or even the truth that I feel like I can't breathe. They assure me my "numbers" are fine as they get me upright. Then, a rag is suddenly stretched across my mouth and I'm laid back into the bed as the water is poured on my face.

> Don't recognize my description? I'm being waterboarded like enemy prisoners of war. Water fills my mouth and nose at the same time, flooding my sinuses and esophagus causing a gag reflex to exhale the oxygen out of my lungs. The cloth around my face prevents any water from escaping. The constant flow of water

prevents me from inhaling or exhaling any further oxygen without aspirating water. Thus, I am tortured with the fear and panic of drowning over and over without the reality of actually drowning.

By the time my therapy session ended, the therapist would straighten the sheets on my bed and put my blanket back on me and call it progress. I was exhausted from the torture and oftentimes left more discouraged than when they started.

Everyday this happened to me, and sometimes twice a day.

Remember that earlier I spoke about not knowing how to pray? I asked God if I was doing it right. On that Monday when I sent out those text messages offering my surrender I had just completed another therapy session. Oh, I wrestled those therapists so good (and raised such a ruckus in doing so) that the nurses' station had to call to ensure everyone was all right. I was worked up and angry. But therapy was over, and the therapists were working to straighten out my sheets, which were wound up tighter than a ball of yarn. They asked if they could stand me up for 30 seconds to fix the bed.

Remember, I was not able to stand at all at this point without a considerable amount of help. Thus, a large male had his hands under my arms in a bear hug to hold me up. I agreed to try so at least I would have a comfortable bed to return to. I pushed as hard as I could with my skeleton legs as I stood next to my bed. The therapist behind me wedged me against the bed, the wall behind me and a walker in front of me. He kept one hand on my chest and used the other hand to assist the other therapist with the sheets.

I felt a light breeze wash over my face ever so lightly and glanced toward the window, but it was still shut. My eyes were suddenly heavy. The tension in my body released as I pushed through the ground with my skeleton legs. I raised up to a normal standing position and closed my eyes as an absolute calmness presided over me. If I had been dying this experience would be absolute comfort. But, I wasn't dying. To the contrary, I experienced an energy light up my body and seem to connect to my mind. I opened my eyes with an inspirational thought: "You are doing it right." I would describe it as similar to the visualization techniques athletes use. I blinked and heard it again: "You are doing it right."

I then noticed there was no chaos in the room, only peace and calm. The main therapist stared at me from the other side of the bed.

Therapist: "Are you okay?"

Me: "Yes."

Therapist: "You look so calm. What changed?"

Me: "I can breathe!"

The second therapist put me back in bed and put the covers on me before they left the room. It took me only a split second to connect what happened.

God had answered my question!

I leave you with this note. Bleomycin toxicity and severe side effects happen to only about 10 out of every 100 chemotherapy patients. Of the 10 patients affected, 9 die due to acute respiratory distress. The remaining 1 person who survives the severe toxicity has symptoms that medical professionals detect before the third infusion.

I took nine infusions of bleomycin. Yet I am alive. God loves me as He loves us all. I am listening. Are you?

CHAPTER THREE

My Linus Blanket

I arrived at the specialty hospital after waking up from the medically-induced coma. I didn't understand the urgency as the paramedics whisked me quickly into a dark storage closet. Enough light seeped under the door for me to see medical equipment surrounding me. LED lights were blinking on equipment near me as I tried to focus my eyes. I could not move any of my extremities. My eyes filled with tears as I understood that had I messed up again. How could I continue to do stupid things and face punishment yet again? Before I could give it much thought, I heard the following conversation:

Nurse: "Do you know where you are?"

Me: "Yes."

Nurse: "Where?"

Me: "A jail in Juarez, Mexico."

It turns out that nothing in the paragraph above is true. After talking to people who witnessed my admission to the specialty hospital, I realize that this was just a hallucinated interpretation of events.

Odd how the mind works. To get a sense of the reality of my situation, imagine going to sleep in a hotel room on your first night of a business trip and waking up six weeks later with these limitations:

+ In six weeks, you missed out on holidays, birthdays, and major sporting events and you don't even realize it.

+ You cannot talk, so no one thinks to tell you what happened to you starting with the fact you are two months ahead on the calendar.

+ You have a tube connected to your throat that leads out to a computerized device that makes a noise you could almost fall back asleep to as white noise.

+ You cannot move your hands, arms, or feet due to muscle atrophy.

+ You have nerve damage along the entire right side of your body that causes enough pain to make you wonder if you had a stroke.

+ You get only rare glimpses of the sun in the small dark room. Are you getting a sense of my reality of that situation?

+ Hospital staff moved in and out, and some simply ignored me because my "numbers" were good and they couldn't be bothered to try to read lips or wait for me to point to pictures of questions I might need answered. Meanwhile, the bills still needed to be paid, and my employer did not go out of its way to help. Oh, and just think how many passwords to your electronic devices and accounts you would end up forgetting!

All of these things caused me intense anxiety that was overwhelming, filled with strange faces and sharp objects, loud noises, and lack of oxygen. I experienced an emotional anguish that required a comfort object to help control my emotions and cope with the trappings of a chaotic world.

My prayers for such a comfort object were answered by an organization that makes blankets for patients. I was not a specific patient and knew no one, and yet I received a blanket made of blue-and-white tie-dye fleece with knotted tassels around the borders. The blanket provided me with comfort and warmth. I often wrapped myself in it the way a mother swaddles a newborn child. The blanket became my go-to-sleep companion, my stress relief, and my best friend. It became known as my Linus blanket.

My Linus blanket offered me comfort in my life's storms. I rubbed it against my cheeks. I folded it and placed it over my eyes, luxuriating in its soft, smooth texture when I felt alone in the hospital. So there I was, confined to a hospital bed with the quiet philosophical wisdom of a grownup, all the while holding onto a beloved remnant of my childhood.

Oh, sure, I received plenty of comments about my Linus blanket from family, friends, and staff. But, even though their laughter was at my expense, they were the first to straighten the blanket out for me at night or after an exhausting therapy session. When it needed washing, I only allowed it to be shaken out in the room. If you thought it was a miracle when Jesus walked on water, then you would witness a true miracle indeed if anyone had dared try to escape with my blanket because I was prepared to race out of bed and tackle. As if I didn't have anxiety over many legitimate issues, when it came to my Linus blanket I was like a 3-year-old boy with his hands on the washer the first time it got washed after I got home, watching to ensure the gremlins didn't snake my blanket through the water drain. I only had one simple rule: *No one was to use my Linus blanket but me!*

So, to fast-forward to the present day: I slowly transitioned from the physical blanket to my faith in God's Security Blanket of Love. This blanket is wrapped around my heart for comfort, around my head and body for protection, and around my life for purpose. It cools me from life's unbearable heat of pain and distress. I take comfort in knowing it has passed every test mankind has imposed on it throughout the centuries. It reminds me that my sickness is not a punishment from God but merely an effect of original sin. My disease, and all our diseases, are a part of the human condition. We are all susceptible to illness, and some of us suffer more illness than others. My local priest explained this perfectly.

Me: "Did this happen to me because I have sinned?"

Father: "Would you punish your own sons to the point of great pain and suffering?"

Me: "Of course not."

Father: "Do you love your sons more than God loves you?"

Me: "No."

Father: "Then why do you think God would punish you?"

Enough said! God's Security Blanket warehouse is overflowing with inventory. Please help yourself to one.

MIRACLE OF AN ORDINARY GUY

CHAPTER FOUR

Spoken Words

I know you don't know this, but I can hear you. The word "worried" does not even begin to describe your emotions. A coldness chills your heart due to a feeling of helplessness. I feel it in your hands as you cup them around my hand underneath the blanket. Your words are whispered and yet I hear them as loud as church bells in a tiny village.

"I'm here. I won't leave you. I love you. Please come home."

I can see you standing next to me staring over the top of my head watching the lights on the monitors. I don't know what all the numbers mean either, but if they are beeping then my heart must be pounding. Keep talking to me, I beg you, but my lips don't move.

My spirit lifts and I hold you. Close your eyes and breathe. I'm here. Feel me wrap around your body and share life's heavy burden of stress. Jesus is with me. He says it's okay if I share the load with Him and carry you through this trial. So much love is being poured into you right now, yet you feel only sorrow and weariness. Don't you remember how happy you were as a teenager pretending to help me put up the swimming pool in your backyard? I'm not sure if either one of us actually knew what we were doing. Your dad got the biggest surprise. Instead of getting a pool, he got a son-in-law ... for 27 years and counting.

It's funny how I can see you so clearly as you stare at me with tears in your eyes. I'm sad as a tear escapes your eye and slowly runs down the side of your cheek. You tried to wipe it away, but it falls and hits my arm evaporating into my bloodstream and invigorating my energy. I'm fighting for you. I try to blink to get your attention. My eyes are so heavy. I can't open them despite how hard I try. Come rest your head on my chest and cry. I was wrong all these years. It is okay to cry in front of others. Being strong is not defined by whether or not you shed a tear. You do not need to be fearful of what others think. They understand and have more love for you than you realize.

> "I'm here. I won't leave you. I love you. Please come home."

Jesus tells me we are blessed with so many guardians. I try to explain that we don't come from a big family and concentrate on raising our children versus sharing time with friends. He puts His hand on me to remind me that we are all His Father's children. My friends and your friends and our family's friends have turned into a prayer chain reaching around the world, spanning multiple ethnicities and religions. There is so much love and kindness in the world, and yet you are sad, afraid, and alone.

I hear your footsteps walking away and fear you are leaving and will not return to me. You are achingly tired. Your eyes are heavy from lack of sleep. You feel the weariness in every joint as you move around the small room trying to sit, stand, and even recline in the chair. Despite the tiredness, you are kept awake by the torment in your mind — if there were something more that you could be doing or some flaw in the choices being made. You record all you can in a spiral notebook, not sure if any of it really makes sense.

I am shouting at you, but no words come out. I've learned that the more excited I get I can make the monitors announce my need for attention. The problem is that it brings a crowd of people into the room. Don't they understand I just want a few minutes alone with you to say everything will be okay? You explain to the nurses that you lay in bed all night waiting for the phone to ring with bad news until the alarm clock finally rang at 5:30AM. You rushed through a shower before the circus act of getting the boys up, dressed, fed, and out the door to school. The boys don't seem to ask many questions about Dad. How would you even begin to explain?

The staff dissipates slowly from the room. It's amazing how someone in a coma can create such havoc. I sense we are alone again only to see you on your phone. So many updates to give out. There has to be a better system as everyone wants an individual report, and by the time you are finished, the first person is calling back to find out if there have been any changes. After answering all the messages, you decide to take a quick picture of me. I quickly try to reach your arm so I can ask you if you remember our prom picture from 1986 when I not only had hair but the big comb in my back pocket to work it. And what about our wedding picture?

Those were happy photos. This one will not show my best side. I don't recognize myself now as I have two poles holding 9

IV pumps each with a line entering my skeletal body of 144 pounds, compared to the 202 pounds I weighed when I was admitted — just three weeks ago! The good news is that I know I'm not in Heaven yet because I'm still wearing this gown that looks like the back of a poker card.

You lay your phone down on the bed and touch my face. This is the hard part of each day — saying goodbye. The hour is getting late and the boys still need a mom. How do we part ways even briefly when nothing in life is guaranteed? Come and let me give you comfort with a hug. But my body still doesn't move! For all I know, you don't hear a word I'm saying. I feel your loneliness. I hear you tell me that I don't say much, but the house is a bit colder and darker without my presence.

When you are all packed up and run out of excuses to stay, you softly whisper the sentences:

> "I'm here. I won't leave you. I love you. Please come home."

Well, my love, I am home now and truly awake! I heard your spoken words the entire time!

CHAPTER FIVE

Random Thoughts on Hospitalization

† No matter how long you stare at the calendar, you cannot go back in time.

† There is more to me than is written in the chart or notes. Get to know the whole "me." I might just surprise you with displays of hidden strength and courage.

† Please write the day of the week where the patient can read it. Every day ends in "y" and over an extended time it is hard to track over whether it's Tuesday or Thursday.

† Personalize your hospital room, especially for extended stays, as the cost of that reclining chair is so much more than any 5-star hotel room. Bring in a collage of family pictures, a handmade blanket, or even a miniature fan to give you a sense of personal space.

† Remember that you are also paying for the bed. Don't let past barriers prevent you from crawling

up into bed with the patient. That is often very encouraging as it creates the right amount of positive energy needed in the healing process.

✝ If the hospital staff ever offers to take you for a walk outside, accept the offer. I remember being wheeled outside for the first time in more than three months and experiencing sensory overload. I smelled the time of day, the fresh cut grass, and the flowers recently planted. I heard the birds chirping when no one else bothered to notice. I saw the vibrant colors of green grass, maroon tree leaves spitting furry white flakes into the air, and bright yellow day lilies. The breeze touched me like an angel welcoming me back to the outdoors.

✝ The way a person enters the room can affect the patient's mood and recovery either *positively* or *negatively*. If you don't introduce yourself or immediately start banging items around in the room as if life is a rush, we quickly burn up our energy in fight-or-flight response.

✝ Good doctors don't just tell you what you need to do; they make you *believe* you can do it.

✝ If your accredited protocol or Magnet status does not match *my* status or illness, please find one that does instead of forcing my square peg into your round hole. Adam and Eve's fingerprints taught us that no two things are ever alike. I am an enigma of complicated problems, so please be good at solving puzzles.

✝ When I pressed the call button, the good nurses and support staff knew it wasn't always my body that needed attention — sometimes my mind needed calming, or my heart needed soothing, or my hand simply needed to be touched. Personally, I loved having my hand held. The truly great ones actually laid down their "professional" shield and sat on the edge of my bed and listened.

✝ After hospital discharge, life moves fast — faster at times than best intentions. I like to believe that most patients, like me, come to feel during our hospital stay that all the doctors, nurses, CNAs, therapists, and the entire support staff are a bit like family. It's amazing how close you can become to one another only to separate one day and never see one another again. It's like a separation or divorce. If we don't come back, it doesn't mean we didn't love you for the care you provided. It might be as simple as not having a ride or not wanting to expose our weakened immune system to the "risky" hospital environment.

✝ If I'm in a medically-induced coma, please talk to me. I can hear you. It might not be in the same context as if you were standing at my bedside having a conversation with me, but the message will be delivered. I can only speak from my experience. I had dreams or hallucinations due to the drugs they administered to stabilize my health. More than four months after waking, I would hear loved ones say certain phrases and sentences and instantly recall hearing them when I was in a coma.

✝ Medically-induced comas can produce both happy and terrifying dreams. I would like to think that happy stories shared by loved ones and friends can have a positive influence. Also, play soft, relaxing music for me to listen to when the room would otherwise be quiet.

✝ Repairing the human spirit is equally as important to healing as repairing the physical ailment. If you wouldn't tell a person with a compound arm fracture to "just rub some dirt on it," why would you think it okay to tell a patient with anxiety issues to "just relax." Neither method works.

✝ When the patient's spouse is in the room, don't treat him or her as invisible. Take the time to explain procedures and medications. We didn't know that ARDS stood for Acute Respiratory Distress Syndrome nor how critical it was. Another example was the ventilation weening protocol, until finally a newly assigned respiratory therapist finally sat down with us and wrote out the methodology used to ween a patient off equipment.

✝ Keep a journal of events for the patient to read after leaving the hospital. I wanted to know every detail of what happened both medically and family-wise while I was sleeping.

✝ The main support person(s) needs as much love as the patient. Loneliness and despair can be a tough enemy to face. A sick child often has parents to comfort each other, but what happens when it is one of the parents, a single parent, or separated parents? Life continues despite the extended hospital stay. Volunteer to help and support the support person knowing that it is tough to accept help and even harder to ask.

✝ Pay Attention ~ Give Love ~ Listen ~ Say Nothing and Hug

✝ The Army calls them "After-Action Reviews," which are deep surveys of what worked and what didn't work after an operation or battle. My therapists did a great job of taking me from a slug with no coordinated muscle tone to a functional human person, but when I got home I found a laundry list of tasks I wasn't prepared for such as simply pushing my wheelchair on carpet. I suffer from respiratory distress, so the added friction from the carpet turned out to be a major obstacle. It would help if a social worker arranged an after-action review meeting a week after discharge to discuss what went well and lessons learned for the patient. The information they gathered could be a huge help for other patients and their families.

✝ Someone please help with insurance companies. After I was discharged from the hospital life was no longer sheltered but fast again. Bills needed to be paid and family/friends needed to return to work. I don't have the descriptive phrases to describe how utterly exhausted I was trying to manage my compromised condition against an employer unwilling to help and an insurance company in the "deny all first request" mode. That battle was almost as great as the fight against cancer. Perhaps one of my readers can explain why we pay premiums — ridiculous!

✝ Please do not wear perfume or bath lotions as both can be difficult for patients, especially respiratory patients — to inhale. Though this should be obvious, respiratory therapists were the worst offenders.

✝ Patients aren't the only ones who need success stories. Doctors and nurses need success stories, too. Take the time to say "thank you" to them after you are discharged. It will mean the world to them.

✝ Sometimes I don't need you to fix my problems — just please let me voice my frustration on how much this disease sucks!

✝ Are you comfortable with me shedding a tear in front of you? If not, it only means I am crying alone.

✝ If at all possible, let us wear our own clothes. I cannot find the words to describe the feeling of putting on my own t-shirt for my last 5 weeks of hospitalization. My self-esteem sky-rocketed to the point it had a positive effect on my therapy sessions. I felt like a person again rather than a specimen.

✝ Life is a gift. Keep in mind that some gifts are better than others.

✝ Even the greatest success stories begin with a single step.

To everyone who provided me care and love during my hospitalization: THANK YOU!

MIRACLE OF AN ORDINARY GUY

CHAPTER SIX

Don't Become a Label

I heard the soft knock on the door as I always asked for the staff to leave it cracked. I battled my body's inability to regulate my core temperature with the room thermostat. If the door remained closed, icicles actually formed on the ceiling, and I found myself covered in the Linus blanket too cold to eat my meals without shivering. If the door was left open, the room got hot and I was overwhelmed with the rush of noises from the hallway.

"Come in," I said from my bed, as I had a thousand times before this occasion. I expected to see the nurse or CNA checking on me, but instead another patient used his walker to enter the room. He appeared to be average height with a trimmed beard flecked with hints of gray. He was in a hospital gown but had a light cloth over his head that extended down around his neck and shoulders. He gripped the walker strongly with calloused hands, telltale signs of his work in the trades in previous times. The walker had a basket attached to the front containing a plastic bag filled with a towel. He spoke first.

   Patient: "Do you mind if I enter your roof?"

I thought it was an odd question and slid my hand to the nurse call button as I responded.

Me: "Sure. What can I help you with?"

The patient came in, and I could see that he appeared to be of Mediterranean descent, which could explain his unique way of asking permission to come in. He walked to the side of my bed and motioned to the chair.

Me: "Yep, I guess… Have a seat."

The patient turned away from the chair and reached a hand back to grab the chair arm and slowly lowered himself to a seated position. He moaned slightly as he reached to turn the walker so he could remove the bag.

> **Patient:** "I'm not sure if you recognize me, but I am in the therapy room watching as everyone struggles to do what others take for granted. You have a gift, you know?"

Me: "I'm sorry. I don't think I follow you."

> **Patient:** "I once experienced a suffering far greater than what I suffer now. Now is simply a fact of my body getting old and worn out. It has provided me many good years in my travels. I learned in my suffering the goodness in people and the need to reset your compass in life to maintain the proper course. You are doing good things here as I see your enthusiasm for your recovery and the motivation for others to emulate. I wanted to share with you a token of my kindness and love."

I watched as the patient reached into the plastic bag and removed a towel with something rolled up inside of it. He gently unrolled the cloth and removed a flat piece of bread.

Patient: "This bread is made in my bakery and I want to share it with you. Please, will you accept a piece of my bread?"

The patient ripped the flat bread in half and handed it to me. I reached out and accepted the bread as I looked at the patient. It was neither hot nor cold, but the texture was soft like toast. I'm not accustomed to accepting goods from strangers. I guess all my years in police work left me somewhat cynical. But things were different as I felt as though I had known this guy all my life.

Me: "Thank you."

As I took the first bite, the patient smiled and ate the other half. He stood up and placed the remaining bread back into the towel, rolled it before returning it to the plastic bag.

Patient: "God bless you. I have others to visit tonight, but I'm sure I will see you often."

I finished the bread as I watched him leave the room. I calmly noticed my usual breathing difficulties had subsided and felt a peaceful energy flowing through me. I was still chewing when another knock came on the door. I assumed the patient had forgotten something in the room, but it was the lady volunteer from the church who had provided my communion the previous two days. The lady looked directly at me with no clue as to what had just transpired.

Volunteer: "I see you just received communion. Would you like to say a prayer?"

Our Lord works in mysterious ways far beyond our comprehension. Is it not possible we have encounters such as the one I described above every day and yet fail to have the faith to believe? The encounter above did not actually physically happen, but it did in my prayers. I allow myself to envision and feel His presence by oversimplifying the fact Jesus showed up carrying groceries and asked if He could enter my heart. Thus, I could do my part and accept His invitation to His Kingdom. I let Him in and dined with the Lord in a meal of faith.

Let me give you something to think about.

"Doubting Thomas" earned his label in eight short days. Thomas watched from a distance on Good Friday as Roman soldiers nailed Jesus to the cross. As Jesus' life drained away, so does Thomas' hope. On Saturday, he was in shock. On Sunday, Thomas was so disillusioned that he did not gather with his fellow disciples for an evening meal. On Monday, the disciples found Thomas and told him, "We have seen the Lord." But Thomas said to them, "Unless I see the mark of the nails in his hands and put my finger into the nail marks and put my hand into his side, I will not believe." By the next Sunday, Jesus again appeared before the disciples, including Thomas. Jesus said to Thomas, "Put your finger here and see my hands, and bring your hand and put it into my side, and do not be unbelieving, but believe." Thomas answered and said to him, "My Lord and my God!"

But which Thomas do we remember? The disciple who is credited as the first to put into words the public truth that Jesus is both Lord and God or the one who is known simply as "Doubting Thomas"?

The same can be asked of myself when diagnosed with cancer. Will I allow myself to be smothered in self-pity, or will I continue to believe that all God creates is good? Will I slip into a state of depression, or will I trust that God knew me before I was created and has a destiny for me greater than this disease? I only have to remember that God gave us our lives. God gave us our abilities, our talents, our families, our friendships! God has blessed us abundantly.

Cancer provides an excuse for us to allow others to label us as "the guy down the hall with cancer" or "the guy with cancer wasn't at church" or we do it ourselves by saying, "You know me; I'm the guy who was just there in the wheelchair with cancer." It is a constant fight not to let ourselves be defined by the illness we have but rather to retain the path God set us upon to travel.

Do not allow yourself to be known as the "Doubting Thomas."

If you waste a day, then you have wasted the most precious resource we have — the gift of life!

- ✝ Every day we get… *we don't get back!*

- ✝ How we live today… *matters!*

- ✝ How we take the opportunity of today… *counts!*

God has positioned each of us uniquely in this life to make a difference by what we say and what we do. We have a choice — to be a part of God's plan or to be a part of a label. Live your life at full power. This gift of life God has given us is precious, holy, and worth living for today. Live your gift of life to the fullest and be a gift to others. Don't be a label!

MIRACLE OF AN ORDINARY GUY

CHAPTER SEVEN

Miracle for an Ordinary Guy

oday I learned that my cancer went full circle — from stage IV contamination of my entire upper torso to complete remission. The shock I experienced a year ago when they first announced the invasion of cancerous cells and today when they announced the cancer is now complete nothingness has left me speechless and in awe. I am left questioning how this thing called life works. There is no blueprint showing our destination or path to the golden gates of Heaven, but I have to think an ordinary guy like me experienced a miracle. Is it so easy to say the cancer remission is the result of an extremely powerful dose of drugs rather than the intervention of God's love?

I offer you this thought. God has a destiny for me greater than this disease. If remission was all I needed to cure the cancer, then the events of February 25 — when the chemo devastated my body — hold no meaning. I do not believe God punished me or made me even sicker. That is the human condition — having a human body and the human experience. Remember, however, that God created us in His likeness with intelligence, reason, and free will. He used my illness to teach me how to be loved unconditionally by letting me experience…

✝ the soft touch of a caring hand when I can't open my eyes and need to be calm

✝ the voice of a loved one talking to me while I am in a coma not knowing I am hearing every word

✝ doctors challenging their colleagues to save a life out of love

✝ the nurses who patiently listened to me when I couldn't speak words

✝ the respiratory therapists who comforted me by adjusting vent settings or giving me oxygen even when the "numbers" said I was fine

✝ the CNAs who changed my clothes and brushed my teeth as though I was a family member and not a grown adult who could not care for himself

✝ the cleaning ladies who have a heart of gold and know a clean room is a sterile room

✝ the physical therapists who never gave up trying to make my body parts strong and functional again, teaching me the mechanics of transferring from bed to chair

✝ the occupational therapist who used brute strength to lift me to a standing position when I absolutely refused to cooperate because he understood what was best for me

✝ the speech therapist who taught me how to swallow and eat and never lost confidence when I failed the first couple of times

✝ the home therapists who loved me from day one and continue to find creative ways to get me stronger

God also taught me how to love unconditionally and inspired me to write the following poem to share my love:

For you...

You say I should write about my experience so others can understand.

I do not because I know you will drop everything to be by my side.

You say to share my thoughts to allow myself to grieve.

I do not because I know in a heartbeat you would suffer the pain for me.

You say to show emotions so others can see the pain and you are human.

I do not because I never want this to be about me.

You say "why not me and not you."

I say the Lord chose me because you are the better person to guide me through the struggle.

You say you have not done enough.

I say you have done more than I could ever expect.

You say what can I do now.

> I say do what you have always done for me — pray and love me!

Lastly, I received the Anointing of the Sick after my discharge from the hospital. I had the opportunity to celebrate the Sacrament of Penance and Reconciliation to confess my sins and receive absolution. I also received Holy Communion. These three Sacraments provided me with the spiritual and physical strength to renew my relationship with God.

I also received a most gracious gift — one that changed the way I prayed, the assurance that it was okay to pray for myself and to ask the Lord to heal my sickness knowing that He is close to those who are suffering. When we are sick or too tired to pray, the prayers of others keep the Lord at our side and draw on His desire for us to have life.

Renew your vow to pray for those you love and for the strangers whose paths you cross for reasons God alone knows.

I am alive because of prayers, and each of you has witnessed a miracle to an ordinary guy!

CHAPTER EIGHT

Baby Steps

I don't feel any better than I felt a week ago when I found out my PET scan revealed no cancerous activity. I still cannot breathe. My body shows signs of oxygen deprivation with clubbing of finger nails, nasal drip from the exertion brought on by a simple act of brushing my teeth, and speaking in seven-word sentences so people don't detect my breathlessness.

I still have pain. Neuropathy pain can grow slowly within you because it's turned on in varying degrees of tension throughout the day. The pain is kneaded into my central nervous system from my legs in the morning to the diaphragm by lunch and finishing with neck pain around the time the boys get home from school.

And I still have anger. I'm on so much medication for anxiety and depression it seems anger is the only feeling allowed to surface. The boys nit-picking each other as boys do or the loudness of a crowd of people unsettles my nerves. It creates chaos in my mind.

Simply put, I am hurting!

A sliver of a tear formed in my eyes as I sat in the back of the church this past week. My mind wandered from the homily to thinking about the Thanksgiving Day turkey. I get a lot of enjoyment from preparing the turkey with a buttered coating and seasoned rub, the inside filled with dressing. I also cook a second turkey breast in the deep fryer. Yes, there are plenty of leftovers, but protein is beneficial to me. The problem is, I can't carve either bird. I cannot stand and do another task such as carving a knife into the turkey. It takes so much effort to think how to breathe when standing that it limits any fine motor skills.

In 13 months, the treatment used to fight against cancer ended up stealing away my youthfulness. I am doing my best to redefine the new normal for me. It cannot be the carefree guy who coached baseball and basketball for his sons so they could have a familiar face on the field with them to overcome their shyness. It cannot be the adventurous guy who packed up the camper and walked miles in the woods because that was the only way to reach a good hunting spot in public areas. It cannot be the surprising guy who bought porch chairs on Mother's Day because in order for it to be a surprise I would actually need to buy and load the chairs without her help.

What have I become? I don't know the answer... But here is what I do know.

I've spent the majority of my waking moments from over the past several months determined to understand what happened back in February 2016 so I could fix the problem. To borrow the old cliché: my lungs are the peeled lemons in life. They leave a sour taste in my mouth when I struggle to do a task only to find it interrupted by the lack of air. I spend so much time researching bleomycin, clinical studies, and alternative medicine, all in hopes of improving my lung function. But the truth is: It is only when I come to terms with the fact I cannot fix my lungs that I will begin to make my lung lemonade.

I can honestly say it is easier said than done. I am not asking myself to give up hope, just to channel the energy into something I can control and line up with God's plan for me. I do see glimpses of this positive channeling through writing, as I can help someone have a better day or plant the seed in a caretaker's actions to make them a better doctor, nurse, or CNA. I spoke in previous blogs about living each day to its fullest. For me, this means restoring the balance of a healthy body and a blessed soul.

I can control both the body and soul by looking in the rearview mirror at each progressive step towards recovery. I cannot see improvement from yesterday or even last week, but as I look at the past six months, I can measure my strength and progress objectively as follows:

MAY 2016	NOVEMBER 2016
I couldn't use my fingers and barely moved my hand by means of the whole arm.	I have fine motor skills to write, text, and type.
I can barely hold onto an 8-ounce bottle for dumbbell curls.	I do 3 sets of 20 reps using and 8-pound dumbbell.
My life depended on a ventilator to take breaths for me and supply oxygen sometimes equal to 10L.	I rest independent of any medical devices such as a ventilator or CPAP mask. I use a nasal cannula for 3L of oxygen.

MAY 2016	NOVEMBER 2016
I depended on people to read my lips or patiently wait while I wrote things on paper.	Much to the dismay of my children, I have a command voice again to announce it's Saturday chore day.
I didn't eat a meal for more than 10 weeks. I received all nutrition through a stomach tube.	I eat dinner meals with the family, while being able to regain weight the cancer treatment stole from me.
The CNAs used a green sponge to brush my teeth with a formula that tasted like some-one liquidized a car air freshener.	I stood at the sink in November and used the toothbrush and cup of water to rinse the toothpaste from my mouth.
I used a catheter to urinate and a bed pan or the sheet for any bowel movements. The clean-up process was like holding my head under water because I couldn't tolerate any movement.	I can sit at an ADA toilet and actually read the newspaper if I choose to do so. This isn't an easy task as I progressed from the speed round of dropping pants, bowel movement, wipe, and pull up pants in less than 2 minutes because I couldn't breathe otherwise.

MAY 2016	NOVEMBER 2016
I had no strength to lift my arms above my head to shave.	I regularly shave myself at the kitchen table progressing to standing in front of the bath-room mirror.
I required sponge baths that did not happen at regular intervals for 4+ months. I took my first shower in July in a wheelchair because I was too weak to sit or stand.	I take regular showers using an ADA chair, but enjoy the sensation of running water splashing across my face for sometimes as long as 5 minutes. Feels like Heaven.
I absolutely could not sit at the edge of the bed with my feet flat on the floor and back straight for more than a minute.	I sit comfortably on my front porch chair waiting for my children to get off the school bus.
I absolutely could not stand and felt completely helpless when trying to push through my legs to get upright. I was like Jell-O in adult clothes.	I walked without any assistance for over 100 feet, while having a conversation.
I received hugs.	I give hugs.

I now understand some of life's greatest challenges are within us. Life is a battle — a constant fight just to hang in there and not allow "life" to beat you. Maybe you are consumed with illness and your fight is mustering every ounce of energy to get one foot out of bed to the floor. Maybe you have little kiddos and your fight is to get them into bed. Maybe you are fighting a job where you get no satisfaction and experience difficult times with co-workers. Maybe you are fighting relationships with family or friends. What is your fight?

Whatever your fight is remember this: The question is never how many times you get knocked down. It is the number of times you get back on your feet.

We cannot quit.

We must fight the good fight.

For it is in the struggle of the fight that we get tougher.

How many accomplishments in your life that you are most proud of were easy? We are most proud of those things that challenged us the most because we discover how much we have grown despite the hardship. We find in the end that the end result — our growth — was worth the sacrifice.

Remember to take baby steps, one foot in front of the other, and breathe. Life is good!

CHAPTER NINE

Doctor, Did You Know?

Doctor, did you know

...you **HURT** me when you didn't conduct my echocardiogram test before you administered my first chemotherapy treatment?

Doctor, did you know

...you **HURT** me when you didn't put in the central line port before you administered my first chemotherapy treatment causing a burn scar up my forearm?

Doctor, did you know

...you **HURT** me when you couldn't admit you didn't know the cause of my severe fluid retention causing permanent scars along both of my shin bones?

Doctor, did you know

...you **HURT** me when you didn't conduct a lung function test before you administered each chemotherapy treatment and caused irreversible lung damage?

Doctor, did you know

...you **HURT** me when you discovered my temperature at 102.6 during infusion and not only told me to use my own Tylenol but sent me home without observation?

Doctor, did you know

...you **HURT** me when you advised me that the most recent CT scan showed no abnormalities, when in fact the report clearly indicated ground-glass opacification (infectious disease showing lung scarring = bleomycin toxicity)?

Doctor, did you know

...you **HURT** me when you couldn't admit you didn't know the cause of my six weeks of fevers that led to my critical illness?

Doctor, did you know

...you **HURT** me when you admitted you didn't have any experience with bleomycin toxicity but failed to warn me of the dangers and, worse, injected them in me without the due diligence on the risks of the drug?

Doctor, did you know

...you **HURT** me when you joked in front of my children that you didn't know if I was alive or not and actually believed flowers would make everything okay?

Doctor, did you know

...you **HURT** me when you promised each day to prescribe medication to help me with four-plus days of insomnia but never actually did, which led me to a deeper state of depression?

Doctor, did you know

…you **HURT** me when you treated my high level of anxiety with the words, "Just relax!" You wouldn't treat a broken arm with words. Why did you think it would work with my anxiety?

Doctor, did you know

…you **HURT** me when you ignored my pleas for help with Post Traumatic Stress Disorder (PTSD) from my near-death experience combined with confinement in a tiny ICU room for three-and-a-half months with limited physical body movement?

Doctor, did you know

…you **HURT** me when you physically grabbed my gown and yanked me out of bed while shouting profanity at me because you couldn't understand that I wasn't like traditional rehabilitation patients who had full lung capacity. You asked for something I physically could not perform. Couldn't you listen to me?

Doctor, did you know

…you **SAVED** my whole experience by walking straight into the exam room and without hesitation giving me an unsolicited hug and whispering in my ear, "I'm glad you made it!" Who does that anymore? My primary care doctor, that's who! His Mom, who lives in India, stills asks and prays for me as though I am family. Thank you for restoring my hope.

To my readers, I only wish today's blog was a work of fiction. It wasn't. The reality is that I am blessed to have family, friends, and supporters who cared for me. It provided me the hope that always conquered any physical pain and suffering. I owe you the world for loving me!

CHAPTER TEN

Every Breath

W hen does the pain subside? When the PET scan returned negative, my cancer status moved to "remission." Honestly, I felt nothing. I had loved ones and friends patting me on the back and offering kind words as they rejoiced in the news. I was very humbled by the outpouring of support I received and yet I had no emotion to join in the celebration. I liken the experience to the feeling I had when nurses asked me to rate my pain on a 10-point scale. I never knew how to answer. I'm not sure if the difficult part was actually differentiating between a 5 or a 6 on the pain scale or between the physical and the emotional pain.

Cancer took a toll on me and my family. I continue to pray and ask God to help me ensure this fight is never selfishly about me. I never fully accepted the initial diagnosis of cancer and now 15 months later I am being asked to pretend it never happened. Some will say this is not what people expect me to do. But how many people celebrate the day they found out they had cancer? My C-Day is October 5, 2015. It is difficult to forget because I am reminded every minute of every day with the effort it takes to draw a breath or take a step hoping to be without pain.

This might be the only time I share the internal pain this illness wrought in its attempt to destroy me. So, please, pay attention and read slowly and try to visualize the description. The physical pain is the easiest to describe. The evil of cancer and its twin, cancer treatment, figuratively placed a glass bottle in each of my lungs and death struck a mighty blow to my sternum. The blunt force initially hurt my chest muscles in the form of fast respirations that stretched my chest wall to full expansion trying to gather air. The blow also crushed the bottles into shards of glass that ripped open the interior of my lungs. Air enters through my nose and causes the glass particles to shift between air pockets. The friction between glass fragments burns through the lining, and I place my hand on my chest to try to calm my breathing. I quickly exhale air because it feels better when the lungs have no air. There is less room for the particles to move, rip, and shred the tiny air sacs. The problem is, my body requires oxygenated blood. My quick exhales provide little time to get this cycle fully completed. So, slowly, dreadfully, I must try another inhale.

How often does this happen? Every breath.

Cancer treatment played a secondary joke on me. The critical care treatment that saved my life resulted in a trade-off of damaging the nerves that carry messages to and from my brain and spinal cord to the rest of my body called neuropathy. Neuropathy impairs my muscle movement, prevents normal sensation in my hands and feet, and causes pain. Lucky for me neuropathy doesn't discriminate. I feel the pain or over-sensitivity throughout my entire body. The right side is worse than the left. I have to compensate for any activities that require balance and coordination. The right calf feels ice cold internally like chilled water running down and forming a block of ice around the ball of my foot. I reach down to wrap my legs in a blanket, but the skin is normal temperature. I would try wool socks, but my bare feet already feel like I have on a shoe that is tied too tight. It is easy to take breaks to massage my legs because my hands are so tremorous that writing or typing are often difficult. It's a bit frustrating when I try to hit the letter "M" and my whole hand slaps the keyboard and I end up with "sjfhjqtbf." The good thing is that the delete button doesn't tear into the paper the way erasers did when we were growing up without computers.

How often does this happen? Every breath.

Emotional damage... Wow. Where do I even begin? I live the alpha and omega with every breath seeking guidance from our Lord, as the serpent attempts to corrupt my thoughts. Let's talk about the battle. There are many wonderful stories published by cancer survivors who speak of conquering the odds once again to appreciate life. These stories are encouraging and inspirational. But let me try to tell the middle portion of their stories — the part not shown in commercials or even in front of family members. I am told my daily portrait has two sides — (1) the public one that shows a confident, recovering cancer patient in rehabilitation and full of life and (2) the private one that is the suffering me.

I allow myself to think I am 100 percent okay as I sit there in my recliner with my legs up and my Linus blanket wrapped around me on 3L of oxygen. It's almost like nothing ever happened — *almost... nothing.* Then I realize I've been sitting here an extra 10 minutes from the point I really needed to use the washroom....

I reach over and turn the oxygen up to 8L. I close my eyes to muster the fortitude for this act of courage as I must overcome severe pain to do an essential task in life. I push off the chair to a standing position while the serpent strikes hard at my right foot trying to trip me. I am aware of the imaginary swollen foot the size of a grapefruit as I feel my lungs ignite with a raw fire in the center of my chest searing into each lung as I take in the higher oxygen setting. I clench my teeth, standing upright, and grab the oxygen cord and take baby steps. I walk the 25 feet to the bathroom like Frankenstein. I enter, turn, and sit. Standing is not an option as the tremors are back and the lack of oxygen to the brain can cause dizziness if I'm not careful. The respirations are high as I struggle to find a position to regain a sense of calm and balance.

I'm telling myself not to ask for help. My family does way too much for me already. The pain is deep enough to cause a tear, but I cannot show weakness in front of the boys. They need a strong father. I wipe my face clear of any anguish and reverse the process and collapse back in the recliner all the while managing the anxiety I have from the fear of suffocation. All this emotional suffering just to go to the bathroom. It's like this to complete any activity that requires energy and effort.

But what about the real emotional pain? For most cancer patients, the experience is more than one stressful event. It's a chain reaction starting with the confirmation of diagnosis, moving to the review of the best strategies to offer the highest probability of remission, then the actual treatment schedule, and finally the completion of treatment. I can argue I managed most of these stress points reasonably well until the events of February 25, when I was no longer in control. I cannot seem to regain my confidence as I routinely hit trigger points such as news stories, movie trailers, loud or banging sounds, or the fear of being left alone that lead to these symptoms:

- † Feeling defensive, irritable, or fearful

- † Being unable to think clearly

- † Avoiding other people

- † Sleeping problems

I continually replay every event and every day since that first surgery when the biopsies were sent to the lab. It's almost like cancer created its own memory bank in my brain that I cannot close the door to. The bank is full of flashbacks and stress. It is a deep, dark vault that is never empty and only awaits the opportunity to invade my active thoughts.

How often does this happen? Every breath.

I am left with the questions *how will this cancer experience define me?* and *how will these symptoms effect my ability to show people who I am?* To help me, I carry a rosary my family bought for me after the previous one, which I had all my life, was accidentally thrown away at the hospital. I rub my finger along the crucifix to remind me that my pain is nothing compared to the suffering of Jesus. He is the Light in my chest reflecting off the glass particles turning something bad like a broken bottle in a sewer gutter to something beautiful like light shining through a stained-glass window to my soul. I continue to put Jesus at the center of my life and see the good and the bad as challenges I need to face.

I started this blog saying it's not about me, but I had to tell my story to help you understand the pain cancer creates in people. Similar to Plato's quote "Only the dead have seen the end of war," cancer will continue to visit past, present, and future patients in one form or another. The battle never ends completely.

The Christmas season is here, and it is a perfect time to think of others and to pray for someone touched by cancer. It might be a family member, a friend, or a stranger. For me, I pray for the children attempting to bring awareness to places such as St. Jude's Children Research Hospital. Behind those smiling faces on those commercials, I know the pain cancer causes to the patient. No parent should ever have the misfortune of having to endure watching their child suffer.

How often should you appreciate your life and the love of others? Every breath!

CHAPTER ELEVEN

Light Is Life!

I got afraid of the dark this past weekend at 1:25 AM. I heard an apparent noise near the fireplace, so I yelled at the dog thinking he was licking his paws. The noise stopped, and I felt a sudden weight on my lap while I sat in the recliner. I reached my arms out to comfort my son asking, "Why are you awake?" There was no one there! I leapt up with my heart suddenly in my throat. I looked around and saw only darkness. I wasn't clever enough to turn on the TV to shine light into the room. I frantically searched to find my flashlight. I am 48 years old and needed to download a nightlight app on my iPad to get me through the night.

One would not need to look far to discover stories about the dualism of light and darkness. This existence of light and darkness has many biblical and spiritual meanings. The definition suggests the two contrasts are made of equal parts. But in reality, they are not equal. Light is something. It can be measured and described numerically in mathematical terms of intensity. It is visible to the naked eye and a part of our everyday experience. It is energy. Darkness, on the other hand, is nothing. It is the absence of light, which makes the measurement of darkness null and void. It has no consequence, effect, or value.

There are times in life when we are in the dark and absorbed in something. It is consuming us. It is drawing out all our energy and taking all our life. It is demanding all the emotion from us and giving nothing in return. It sucks out our soul. Maybe it is anger and rage that have no outlet, expression, or purpose. Maybe it is grief where we are swallowed up in pain along with misery, loss, and loneliness. Maybe it is a fear that keeps gnawing at us like an open sore along with anxiety and doubt. It consumes us and gives us nothing. We are in the dark.

We have become the cartoon character with the rain cloud always hanging over our head taking away life and giving back nothing. These feelings of darkness can happen very acutely. There are times we know it all too well. There are times we wish it weren't so. The human life has experiences that for many of us are very real. They can be very scary and very dark.

But then the smallest measurable particle of light enters our heart. We learned in high school physics that the elementary particle is called a photon. We learned in Christian theology that the elementary light is our Savior. The difference between the two studies is that God is the living being who comes to us in the dark. He comes to us in our rage, in our anger, in our fear, in our loneliness, in our grief, in our loss, and in our anxiety. God comes to us casting out the darkness. He gets rid of the nothing and puts in the light. By His light, all the darkness withers away.

How do we find the light in our own lives? I try to keep it simple. My first prayer is,

> Yes, Lord, I offer my life, and please work through me
> TODAY.

It took me a while to understand that my recovery was my main mission in life and that I could not reverse all the damage I sustained in a single workout. The approach must be to remember that every significant achievement in human history started with something small. These tiny steps add up over time to form a process and grow. Our lives can be broken down into stages, each of which has processes and lessons to learn, so we can be patient and understand that God is in control and allowing it to unfold if we allow it to.

This is an important point, for God gave each of us the power of free will. By definition, free will is the ability to make choices that are not controlled by fate or by God. If we do not pray and trust in God to take our heavy burdens from us, He will allow us to continue to exercise the free will He created in us to make our own choices without His interference. If your problems and fears are not going away, ask yourself if you have surrendered your fears to our Lord without hesitation or doubt.

Once I accepted God's love, I absorbed His light. I answered, "Yes, Lord, I offer my life, and I want to cooperate with Your guidance and strength to become the person You know me to be." I then asked, "Help me TODAY, even if it's in the smallest way, to take the next step." My smallest step was the decision to no longer use the term "sick" when describing my condition. Sick implies a physical or mental illness associated with a disease. I am not sick. Instead, I have "injured" lungs that are damaged from the effects of chemotherapy. I have the determination to work hard, and God's light will restore the muscles and nerve function controlling my physical, sensory, and mental capabilities that were lost due to injury. What I cannot find are the words to describe the feeling of God's love and the overwhelming sense of happiness and energy He allowed me to experience this week.

The second part of finding the light is understanding that it is meant to shine everywhere and on everyone. I now pray,

> Yes, Lord, I offer my life, and please work through me
> to help others TODAY.

Light is meant to be passed on and shared with others like a torch in the darkness. My recovery is steadily improving, and I am ready for the second phase of God's work to help others. I carry the torch knowing I do not need to solve anyone's problems. I wrote in my journal recently about my view on friendship. I would rather have a few who are intimate and reliable than many who are distractible and indifferent.

So, what does this torch look like? It is an unexpected phone call to a troubled person and doing nothing but listening. It is arriving at their door with a bag of groceries because they needed them but were too proud to ask for help. It is a hug, a kind word, a touch of the hand, a hidden note in our child's lunchbox saying "I love you" because it's been a bad homework week. It is sneaking out to fill your spouse's car with gas so they don't have to in the morning because the commute is unbearable most days. It is washing the dishes because everyone enjoys coming home to a clean house. It is being kind to others without asking for anything in return. These things I know because I was the troubled person and God worked through others to brighten my day.

Light gives us new hope, new strength, new grace. Light is a love God gives to us to fill the voids of darkness. The power of light changes lives, transforms hearts, and creates warmth and beauty. We must learn to see not with our eyes, but with our heart. So, find the quietness of the day to slow your heartbeat, feel the rosary beads in your hand, whisper your burdens to the Lord, and ask Him to set you free. Don't merely ask Him to solve your problems and expect a roadmap on the pillow next to you when you wake. If God revealed His plan for each of us, there would be no struggle, no need for emotion because our final destination would be easy to reach by following a GPS. There is a reason we were not born with an expiration date stamped on our feet. God meant for us to walk by His side each day as if it were the last!

MIRACLE OF AN ORDINARY GUY

CHAPTER TWELVE

Listening Is a Skill

G rab a lighter or one of those "flickers" used to light a candle or the grill. Flick it.

See how quickly the flame appears and yet, in an instant, it is gone when you release the button. We take the fire for granted, except when the electricity goes out in a storm and we can't remember where we left the flicker. The flame isn't as easy to create now.

Our faith can be described as the flame. When it is easily available, it is convenient for us to be comforted by its warmth. What happens when an unexpected storm comes? Do you panic when you can't find the flame? Do you quickly point out how chaotic the world has become and begin looking for other shortcuts?

Slow down…and listen. Be still for a moment and shut out all the surrounding distractions. That is not easy to do. How did an ordinary guy turn the radio knob and tune in directly to God's voice? Surely, God did not speak louder to me than any person reading these words. He surely didn't love me any more or less than any other person. The difference is that my body helped me develop my skill for listening.

Let me be crystal clear: God did not create my illness or the events of February 25. Those are the shortcomings of having this human body. If anything, God reminded me He understood suffering. It is something He is close to and He is close to us when we are suffering, even when our minds lie to us telling us that He is very far away.

Here is how merciful our Lord is to us. I was sick weeks before my critical day. I battled to get out of bed, shower, and dress for work. I didn't eat much anymore, so I skipped breakfast and drove the 45 minutes to work. I lumbered up to the 18th floor to sit in my office and watch the race between the clock and the next fever, knowing the body chills would be so difficult to hide because I needed to wear a jacket inside my office to stay warm enough to do my job. I would head home dreading the 90-minute commute and try to eat a dinner. There was no joy to the food. I tried to treat it like a workout. Working out never feels great, but it is essential to stay in shape. In my case, the approach to eating kept my weight level high enough to complete my chemotherapy treatments. I counted down each one, completing 9 of 12. I spent the last bit of energy by changing into PJs and falling into bed. That's it! That was every day of the last three weeks before I went into the coma – except for one 24-hour period.

In the midst of this three-week stretch, I experienced a "break" from my illness and symptoms. I had a fishing trip planned more than six weeks prior to the increased side effects of the chemo treatments. The day started like all others. I sluggishly gathered clothes and showered until 1 PM, then loaded the car for the two-hour trip to Michigan where I would meet a friend and his dad and brother for walleye fishing on the St. Joseph River. As

I loaded the last of my gear into the car, almost immediately I noticed my energy returning to me. I stood in the driveway and felt the cool, brisk air hit against my face and waken me for the drive. The miles went quickly and soon enough I found myself standing in a log cabin built for two that we were going to jam the four of us into. Aside from my friend's dad, the three of us hadn't missed many meals in life so the quarters would be tight. I took a picture of the sleeping arrangement and sent it to the others who were due within the hour to say it was a good thing we had thought to bring the cot because there was only a single bunkbed and a full-size bed. The reply came: "We forgot the cot!"

The good thing about arriving first means you get the first choice of racks. I chose the top rack despite my low energy to climb the flimsy ladder and the mattress just barely as wide as my shoulders. I thought this was a good idea, but seeing how I nearly always went to the bathroom once or twice a night when I wasn't tossing and turning, the choice had *fall* risk written all over it. The other guests didn't think it was a great idea either but couldn't argue another choice since they forgot the cot.

We fished a bit the first night without any luck and drove into town for dinner before returning for a campfire outside the cabin. The entire time I either stood to fish or sat with the others to eat. I lay in bed and marveled at how well I felt. I heard the calm humming of the portable heater and felt an inner peace I hadn't felt in some time. My shoulders hit the ceiling when I tried to turn over, but I didn't have any other problems such as chills, fever, or falling out of bed to pee. In fact, I actually felt like driving home when we woke at 3 AM to fish because I didn't want to lose the moment.

The fishing was slow out of the boat the four of us shared trying not to hook each other in the eye with our casts. The cold air penetrated the multiple layers of clothes, and the mist from the dam didn't help. The good thing about the boat is that the bow contained a plexiglass type enclosure with a heater and a bench on each side. When you got cold, you could duck inside and sit to warm up. I don't think I went inside more than three times before the fishing got heavy at 7:30 AM. For a 20-minute period, the bite was on. We shouted mocking a local fishing program "Get the Frabill" referring to the brand of fishing net. My friend earned his title as 'The Net Man." We hooked six walleyes for the day as I was one of two people still standing and fishing off the back of the boat when our paid time ended. Everyone else sat on the benches inside the warm enclosure.

We split the fillets and packed the car before we said goodbye. I realized during the drive home that I had experienced something I could not describe. I was not in pain. I was not nauseated. I was not fatigued. In fact, I was actually hungry. I stopped and ate an entire 10-piece Chicken McNuggets with fries from McDonald's. It was probably the most I ate at any one sitting in more time than I could recall. I returned home in time for the fevers to start by dinnertime.

I can look back in time and recount exactly how the days' events unfolded as described above, but why couldn't I see the gift of mercy as it was being fulfilled in front of my eyes? I experienced something that I was aware of, but I didn't make the connection between my suffering and God's mercy because I didn't listen to the message. It's not unlike a conversation between two people. We are all busy and bombarded by a multitude of stressors. We use words such as "multi-tasking." Let me stop you with this thought because this was exactly where I was in my life with trying to balance family, treatment, work, sickness, appointments, and friends.

Each one of these entities was requesting time, but here is the simple math. Computers compute hundreds of billions of lines of code in a second. No matter how quickly the computing takes, it is still accomplished a single task at a time. *There is no such thing as multi-tasking.* We consciously decide how much attention we assign to each message. I didn't hear God's message and missed His act of mercy at the time it was happening because I didn't listen.

I treated my faith like the flicker in my hand. When I needed God in my life, I made a conscious effort to connect to Him and tried to listen only when it was convenient to my time line. My hospital stayed slammed the brakes on all distractors in life. Faith became the answer to my fear. The very real chance of death and the fear of God's judgment, the unknown, and not being loved surrounded me. It took that dark storm to release me from my earthly dependencies on "stuff" I thought was important to break down to the point that I actually talked to God and asked Him to relieve me of the darkness. It was only then that I saw the light was not controlled by me like the flame of a flicker. God showed me He was stronger than the darkness by revealing Himself. The flame and the light are Jesus Christ.

The purpose of my writing is self-analysis. It is a forum I can speak from experiences that worked for me. Listening is a skill whether it is a loved one or our relationship with God. When we don't fully commit to the act of listening, we are missing out on building layers of trust and confidence. Where did I start? I started by committing to prayer *every day*. No excuses! If God is the center of my existence, then He is important enough to dedicate time to. Am I good at structured, heartfelt, and purposeful prayer? No! But it's like the old golf tale "all putted balls that stop short of the hole have 0% chance of going in." By not praying at all, I have 0% chance of getting better.

Am I any better at listening to loved ones? No! But, I am trying. God can only work so many miracles on me within a given year!

CHAPTER THIRTEEN

I Gave Him My Heart

Exactly one year ago today, I lay in the ICU room on my back with my head slightly elevated. I wore a re-breathing mask to filter the high flow of 15 liters of oxygen into my lungs. My mind was too exhausted to even begin to analyze the events that had transpired since my admission. In fact, my mind ingested so much medication to sedate me during the intubation time that I blinked my eyelids quite a bit in an attempt to squeeze reality out from the fog of intoxication. I don't remember feeling sad, but worse, I felt close to nothing at all. Feeling required nerves, connections, sensory input. The only thing I felt was numb. And tired. Yes, I felt exhausted.

I had nothing to offer anyone. I lay there defenseless. My life was no more than an exhausted endurance race. Death, who now stood right outside my room, was as familiar to me as a family member returning after a long absence. Every hour on this day a year ago I was asked, "What do you want to do now?" Each time I answered, "I'll keep trying." I believe the nurses knew the right thing to do was to re-intubate me so the ventilator could ease some of the stress being put on my body, but they wanted the decision to come from me.

Death continued to stand at the door awaiting my decision. All my life I measured my success in achievements — education, job positions, leadership accomplishments, house purchases, etc. I thought I controlled my own destiny. Isn't that what we are taught from a very young age starting with our parents. You can be anything you set your mind to. Another thing they instill in us is the saying, "God always has a plan for us."

What happens when the two don't match? I thought I thrived in circumstances where I could control the outcome or at least actively participate. God is always going to allow me to use my free will with the understanding that by exercising my free will and control, I surrender the opportunity for God to work within me. Here's an example: I deal with anxiety issues. I have learned to manage them a lot better, but they are still a part of me. Through prayer, I ask God to take them from me, but I find my anxiety is still here. Is God not listening? No, God is listening. The truth is, I am giving God partial faith. I am only "asking" Him to take the anxiety from me, but I don't trust Him enough to help so I continue to attempt to control the illness. God is not going to intercede in my independence. I have to be "ALL IN." I have to make a commitment to ask through prayer and allow God to do His work without interfering or questioning.

As I became more exhausted as I lay there a year ago, I finally relinquished any thought that I could actually control my outcome. I released my everything to God — my physical exhaustion, my emotional turmoil, and my painful breathing. I focused on the flicker of hope God placed right in the center of my heart. I pressed the call button and asked the nurse to send for the doctor so I could be re-intubated. This seemed like the toughest decision because I did not know if I would ever wake up or if I would sustain brain damage from the lack of oxygen. It didn't take long for the team of doctors and nurses to come in to start the process. I closed my eyes and felt the lone tear spill out of my left eye and run slowly over my cheek. I opened my eyes to see Death walking away. Just then I imaged Jesus standing near me to remind Death that He alone is The Light. What should have been the toughest decision turned out to be the calmest.

Unfortunately, I am speaking only for myself. I felt our Savior's hand cupped over my hand to ensure I knew He was there for me for what seemed like a blink of the eye, but my loved ones sat worried, confused, and sad beyond words as days turned to a week and a week turned to weeks. I wonder if, when they prayed and closed their eyes, Jesus appeared to them in a momentary dream or passing thought to let them know that He was with me. "I'll pray for you" is almost as common a response as "gesundheit" after a sneeze. I don't believe it's possible for humans to fully understand the power of prayer just as we cannot truly understand what the love of Heaven will be like. I do think that you are only talking to yourself if your prayer is not based on a solid foundation of belief and faith.

What I have learned from the year past is something about miracles and prayer — miracles of healing and answered prayer. Each came quietly and simply, on tiptoe, so that I hardly knew it had occurred. All this makes me realize that miracles are everyday things. They are almost routine and yet they are miracles just the same. Every time something hard becomes easier; every time I adjust to a situation that, last week, I didn't know existed; every time a kindness falls softly from an unexpected source; every time a blessing comes not with trumpet and a welcoming party but silently as night, I have witnessed a miracle!

I was wrong when I started the second paragraph with the sentence, "I had nothing to offer anyone." God gave us the ability to choose free will, and so I gave God the one thing He needed from me. I gave Him my heart!

CHAPTER FOURTEEN

Life Lessons from Super Bowl LI

The Super Bowl this past Sunday is being called one of, if not the, most memorable football games in history. Not only was it the first overtime game ever, but it was marked by an impossible-to-believe finish with the Patriots pulling out a stunning victory despite trailing 28–3 with 2 minutes and 12 seconds remaining in the third quarter. If you stayed tuned to watch the comeback excitement — or disappointment if you were a Falcons fan, then you witnessed an example of how the beauty of sports can teach us in compressed time the things we desperately need to know in order to be winners in the game of life.

1. LIFE TAKES PREPARATION TIME.

Team preparations for the Super Bowl centers the maximum synergy between the offense unit, the defense unit, and the special teams unit. By definition, synergy is the interaction or cooperation of two or more elements to produce a combined effect greater than the sum of their separate effects. Similarly, we are constantly attempting to prepare our mind, body, and spirit to achieve peace and happiness.

I try to do this by developing habits that work in favor of the goals I want to achieve in life, then repeatedly practicing them. I do this by establishing a positive daily routine to provide structure and create momentum that will carry me on the days when I feel like I don't have the strength to carry myself. Following a daily routine helps me establish priorities, limits procrastination, keeps track of goals, and even makes me healthier.

Here are a few of the habits I practice:

- † Thank the Lord for a restful sleep and the gift of life.

- † Start the day with a positive quote and visualize a strong mind-body-spirit connection.

- † Try to read a single page of a book before I ever look at my phone or email.

- † Write a daily to-do list consisting of three tasks/activities.

- † Limit the negativity of the news to 30 minutes a day.

- † Get out of my chair…OFTEN! I aim for a walk every hour considering I use only 20 percent lung function; this should be achievable for most.

- † Spend less time with people who don't lift me up. Life is too short to nourish negativity.

2. LIFE REQUIRES CONSTANT EVALUATION AND ADJUSTMENTS.

Halftime found the Patriots down by 18 points. The Patriots had not spent two weeks of game planning and executing during practice only to find the team in this position. But life rarely happens according to our plans. The good teams are able to reevaluate and adjust the original plan of action. I equate my experience to an engine that broke down. The only way to make the machine work again is to break it down to individual pieces, fix the inner parts, and reassemble it. But here's the most important part: Run that engine again at high speed without fear it will break again because you already know if it does it can be rebuilt.

The late Steve Jobs touched on this concept in the commencement address he gave Stanford students by saying,

> "…for the past 33 years, I have looked in the mirror every morning and asked myself: 'If today were the last day of my life, would I want to do what I am about to do today?' And whenever the answer has been 'No' for too many days in a row, I know I need to change something."

Here are a few of the habits I practice:

+ Practice deep breathing and a few minutes of meditation. This helps me to connect with God, to center my positive thoughts, and to check for any symptoms that need adjusting.

✝ I either read or listen to a short five-minute daily prayer. This is about starting my day with God as my focus point as all good things come from Him.

✝ I ask myself three questions:

1. Do I love doing what I am doing?

2. What is the worst that can happen today?

3. What good can I do today?

✝ Journal every task you do in a single day or two days in a row. Then review the list and evaluate the amount of time you are distracted versus productive. You will be amazed as you discover the smallest of activities you can eliminate to reclaim useful time.

✝ If you really want to be creative, add a "mood" emoji next to each activity and use it as a gauge for whether you are having a happy, sad, or somewhere-in-between kind of day.

3. IN LIFE, WE ALL GO THROUGH TRIAL AND TRIBULATIONS.

The Book of Genesis revealed original sin when Adam and Eve ate the fruit from "the tree of the knowledge of good and evil." God punished Adam and Eve by making their lives hard. No longer could they live in the perfect world of the Garden of Eden. Men would have to struggle and sweat for their subsistence. Women would have to bear children in pain. We would forever know about the joy and pain accompanying good and evil along with winning and losing. Trials and distress are not something unusual in life; they are part of what it means to be human in a fallen world.

Here are a few thoughts:

+ Suffering can be a good thing. I do not believe God made me sick, but He did take advantage of my sickness to help me develop a closer relationship with Him.

+ "Blessed is the man who endures temptation, because having been approved, he will receive the crown of life which the Lord has promised to those who love Him" (James 1:12). My sickness asked a very simple question, "Do I have faith in God?" I did not shake my fists at God and ask "Why me?" but instead proved the genuineness of my faith in trial by fire. I survived because I ALLOWED God to let me survive. He is ALWAYS in control, not me. I follow His plan on HIS timeline, not mine.

+ A single friend in a storm is worth more than a thousand friends in a time of calm.

+ It's hard to know the tremendous joys of winning without experiencing the defeats that tore you apart.

+ Sometimes you win and sometimes you learn.

4. CELEBRATE VICTORIES!

It doesn't take a grand event like the Super Bowl to call a day a victory. Victories will happen when you complete the three items on your to-do list that you set out to do in the morning. Victories will happen when you look back in a month and realize you read an entire book because you dedicated reading a minimum of a single page a day before looking at your electronic devices. Victories will happen because you use your shower time to take the cleansing breath and meditate finding our Savior in everything good that surrounds us.

My friends, life is good. Find the strength to see through the fog of the devil's lies that lead to low self-esteem, questioning your faith, and not enjoying the gift of life. It is true: God is in control and has a great plan for each of us. But He granted us free will and the ability to reason. We must decide to be winners like the victors of Super Bowl LI.

CHAPTER FIFTEEN

A Simple Approach to Happiness

I've been practicing smiling lately. Silly, I know. But too many times I heard the sly comment, "You never smile. You always have the straight mouth with no shiny white teeth flashing." So I investigated many of my pictures and concluded that my critics were correct. I never smile. Then I thought deeply on the link between a nice smile and happiness. I concluded that although some things can come into in our lives through luck, happiness is undoubtedly not one of them.

I am interested in being happy. Who isn't? The recovery period during my critical illness gave me plenty of highs and lows ranging from despair to exuberance. It required me to find simple approaches to complete a task by the most efficient means possible. I didn't have a large margin of error. If I stand too long, walk too far, or climb too many stairs respiratory distress will leave my oxygen levels dangerously low. Instead of using a stop watch, I learned to condition myself to accomplish tasks such as brushing my teeth, shaving, or helping with dishes by the number of songs on a playlist. The playlists have been edited each time my body completed a task before the music stopped, sort of like playing musical chairs. If I finished my task and was seated in my recovery chair before the songs ended, then I felt joyful. I always felt happy and satisfied when I made progress. I examined my playlists and discovered that all my songs are filled with consistent messages of goodness.

Could discovering happiness be this easy? The search for happiness is a close second to man's search for the Holy Grail. I took a step back and asked myself specifically what worked for me on days I know I achieved happiness. The answer: Those days I had a clear vision of positive thoughts and beliefs. But any hypothesis needs to be tested before it can be accepted as true. Could it stand up to the smooth goings of life that turn suddenly chaotic or tragic when least expected?

My happiness tools are this simple: Don't Envy, Don't Judge, Don't Blame, and Forgive. Envy is defined as a feeling of discontented or resentful yearning aroused by someone else's possessions, qualities, or luck. I have never in my life envied a human being who led an easy life. Nothing in the world is worth having or worth doing unless it requires effort, pain, or difficulty. Resentment, jealousy, and anger fueled by envy never change another's heart, only mine, because after all, grief often comes from wanting something that isn't ours or that we have no control over.

The ability to observe without judging is the highest form of intelligence. If you spend your time hoping someone will suffer the consequences for what they did to your heart, then you are allowing them to hurt you a second time in your mind. Besides, you never know what others are experiencing within their own lives. I try to recognize that it's okay to disagree with the thoughts or opinions other people express. But just because I don't like what they are saying does not give me the right to accuse them of poorly expressing their beliefs. I do, however, want to be around people who do positive things. I no longer want to be around people who judge or talk about what people do. I want to be around people who dream and support others.

An important decision I made was to resist playing the blame game. Blaming others is an act of refusing to take responsibility for oneself. When I could not accept the fact or the reality, I blamed another person or the situation instead of holding myself accountable. That day in the hospital when I realized that God is in control of my life and knew me before I was even born was the day I began to take control of my happiness. I am in charge of how I will approach problems in my life. "Things" will turn out better or worse because of me and nobody else. That was the day I knew I could truly build a life that matters. I believe it took suffering from an illness to cleanse my spirit to focus on God's gift of life.

I find most often that it is necessary to let things go simply because they are heavy. So, I let them go: I forgive. We have to forgive. We do not have to like the person. We do not have to be friends with them. We do not have to send them hearts in text messages, but we do have to forgive them, to overlook, and to forget. Forgiving is not something I do for someone else. It is something I do for myself. It is refusing to let the past strangle my opportunity to move to the now!

I do recognize life is worth living to its fullest, and it can be summed up simply with a smile. The battles and struggles I face with life's trials and consequences are worth fighting. I remember my faith is a gift that God has given me, not only to give me meaning, purpose, and direction in this life but the beauty and power in Heaven. This is my approach to happiness. It is found in the air I breathe, in my touch, in my words, and always in my smile. Try it for a day and tell me if it makes a difference for you.

CHAPTER SIXTEEN

A Conversation with Me

Q: **How did you find the strength to fight cancer and the damage you sustained from the treatment?**

A: I remember my first fist fight coming in elementary school. The bell rang and I exited the school to head home before I realized I entered a playground cage-match — the cage being the host of student onlookers. I stood toe-to-toe with my foe. This was not a well-choreographed fight scene in a movie or a boxing match with a start bell. No, it lasted less than 30 seconds with a punch to my nose and the world becoming blurry. The yell of an approaching teacher ended the contest, and I resumed my walk home alone. It might have been the first time I had a bloody nose, and I was a bit shocked as I blew my nose and found the blood clotting already as I looked at the mess in the tissue. I didn't cry, but I lost my first battle. There's a lesson here. Every man should lose a battle in his youth, so he doesn't lose a war when he is old. It gave me a taste of defeat that I never wanted to repeat!

Q: Do you get lonely during the day?

A: I do every once in a while, but I try to use the time to free myself from the stress and distractors of life that used to weigh heavily against the equilibrium of my life. I will rebuild myself and return to work. It will take time. My job right now is to heal. I have learned to really sit with loneliness and embrace it as a gift of opportunity to get to know myself, to learn how strong I really am, and to depend on no one but myself for my happiness. I understand now that a little loneliness goes a long way in creating a richer, deeper, more vibrant and charming me.

Q: What was it like to wake up after your medically-induced coma?

A: Surprisingly, I get asked this question more than one would expect. The elapsed time can be measured in a blink of an eye. My experience was similar to going to sleep on a Thursday night and waking up on a Friday morning. I had no idea six weeks were ripped from the calendar. The coma itself carried me into a world where time and space seemed to vanish; it was a dreamlike existence in which people, places, and situations shifted as quickly as thoughts. I had a profound sense of being at a crossroads, a turning point, somewhere between life and death. I experienced the full spectrum of moods from happiness to sheer terror. I have since learned these are all common side effects of the drug fentanyl used to induce the coma.

The actual waking up part found me fighting a cloudy vision of dim lights and shadows of people moving around the room. I did recognize I was in a hospital. My thoughts quickly turned to panic as the complications of muscle atrophy and nerve damage caused the lack of sensation between my mind and body. I thought I was paralyzed because I was too weak to move any of my body parts and the nerve damage made my limbs numb.

The absolute truth is that waking up far outweighs the alternative. It took time for me to adjust to the series of events leading to this next statement: I am a person of faith and belief in God who views my awakening as a blessing to help and inspire others through His Spirit.

Q: What was your life like a year ago?

A: A year ago I was sick. I'm not sure if I couldn't admit it to myself or I simply lost track of the severity of the illness. Either way, I repeated the lie that I was fighting cancer. I think I could only hide the sadness and hurt so much in a smile, before my heart told the truth. I dealt with constant nausea and fevers so that I ached to sleep as an escape because opening my eyes meant waking to a nightmare.

There are no words to explain the pain. It's like a person who jumps from a burning skyscraper. Any person on the ground who shouted in disbelief "Don't!" or "Hang on!" would never understand the jumper. This is because we measure the experience with our own constant variable — fear of heights. However, when a second variable is introduced at the same moment — the terror of the fire's flames, the person jumps because falling to death becomes the slightly less terrible of the two. In the end, you would have to personally battle cancer to really understand the pain beyond just a fever.

Q: How is your life now?

A: Life is good. Let me see if I can get this correct. When I wake to see the light of a new day and the refreshing fragrance of morning, I create a positive thought to begin the journey. I see a new reason to start positivity regardless of the turmoil and trials of yesterday. I demand myself to see a reason to understand and appreciate the real gift of life knowing this could be my last day. I choose positive thoughts over negative thoughts. I find a reason to be happy by breathing a sigh of purposefulness into my actions. I am ready to do something unique and awesome. My only offer of advice to my readers is to find a sense of urgency to live this life to the fullest with love, righteousness, and faithfulness.

Q: What is it like to have anxiety?

A: Anxiety is new for me. I don't remember it being the battle it is for me today before my cancer diagnosis. I think it developed from the shock of feeling healthy with no symptoms and still running four miles a day to learning I was battling stage IV cancer overnight. I added to the plate a near-death experience, trauma of medical staff rushing to my bedside multiple times, being locked in an ICU and isolation room for four-and-a-half months, and accepting a "new" normal for my life. Here's what my anxiety looks like:

- † Being scared to make a phone call or an appointment. It's difficult for me to simply order a pizza.

- † Having a difficult time leaving a voicemail unless I prepare what to say ahead of time.

- † Asking for help at a store.

- † Knowing I am freaking out when there is no reason to freak out, but lacking the ability to shut down the emotion.

I combine my anxiety with Post Traumatic Stress Disorder (PTSD). It is not an illness or disease. I have been through multiple traumatic situations, and this is the effect. I have good days and bad days, sometimes within the same day. Sometimes I have thoughts or memories of my ordeal I would rather not remember. This is something I didn't ask for, but I need to be aware of it. I try to make it through each day by controlling it without letting it control me. The easiest way to deal with me is by giving me your love, kindness, and patience.

Q: Do you have any hobbies?

A: It should be no surprise that I have developed a love for writing. Though I freely admit that I grew up with qualities of being analytical and calculating, while sacrificing creativity, I am often inspired by the Holy Spirit to give me a glimpse of God's message to share. I often ask God to deliver on Mondays to give me the week to work on it, but I waited until Friday night to hear His message. I think He is always reminding me not to get ahead of myself, and I am on His timeline.

Q: What are your future goals?

A: First, to live life to its fullest by living in the moment. Yesterday is gone, and the future is not promised. The moment doesn't have to be defined by grandiose plans such as skydiving and topping Mount Everest. The moment can be putting down the cell phone to give our loved one an unexpected hug to show our love for him or her.

Second, I vow to work hard to repair my body to the best I can control. I cannot will myself to regenerate lost lung tissue. The damaged cells are the "new" me. What I can control is the development of muscle surrounding my lungs to better support my body and learning better breathing techniques to control my diaphragm to maximize the use of the air I do get into my lungs.

Lastly, I would like to give back to others. I had such a positive response to the presentation I gave to our church parishioners that I would like to extend my offer to hospitals and colleges to present my experience as a learning tool. I also think there is room for counseling and group counseling for people experiencing similar experiences.

Q: Last question. Is there anything you wish to add for your readers that I didn't cover in this interview?

A: I want to reiterate the number-one goal of my writing — to help my family and friends to remember the memories this experience brought to us. I hope my family can read or listen to my stories and remember who I am. I hope it always brings warm smiles to their faces knowing the love I have for them.

I defied the odds by surviving the most gruesome battle anyone could have predicted. I no longer fear these smaller daily battles because they are nothing compared to the victory I declared in April 2016 when God sent me back to fulfill His plan. Any obstacles my enemies have for me are nonsense to me because they don't know what I already achieved. I love my readers — those who have followed my blog —— who stood behind me during the toughest times and now enjoy my rekindled spirit to live.

I am a warrior!

CHAPTER SEVENTEEN

God Is Not the Mother Duck!

"For nothing will be impossible with God."
(Luke 1:37, NRSVCE)

I watched a program about animal behavior on the National Geographic channel. The high-definition picture displays such eye-popping colors to entice you to watch even this particular episode, which was on ducks. Interestingly, the program showed the mother duck jumping down into small stream followed by each of the ducklings. They swam around until the mother duck decided it was time to go and leaped to the shore and began to waddle off. One by one the ducklings followed suit with some requiring a second or third attempt to get to shore until at last a single duck remained in the water. Exhaustion settled in as each attempt resulted in shorter gains up the ravine edge. The mother duck continued moving forward. The narrator summarized this as typical duck behavior. The mother duck, taking the last duckling's inability to fly to safe ground as evidence that it was too weak to survive life, therefore abandons the last duckling.

The episode made me think of all our struggles in life and how some of us reach our last attempt to get up the ravine edge and slide back into the frigid waters — all alone. We often seek help in the obvious places as a doctor writes us a prescription or a priest offers a prayer on our behalf. But it's the friend who surprises us and jumps down into the water. We sometimes explode at what seems to be a foolish act until our friend calmly answers that he or she has been in our place before and knows the way out.

Friendship is easy in calm waters. When my body betrayed me and left me alone in the dark, I watched the doorway for my friends to rescue me. Most never showed! The people who did show did so because God put them in my path before I was even born. I might not have understood the purpose until this moment. Unlike the mother duck, God does not abandon us ever — no matter how weak or ill-equipped to survive we seem to be. His love is unconditional.

If our faith reassures us that God's love for us is unconditional, then how do we reach Him when we need Him the most? I think the closest we can humanly imagine unconditional love is the bond between parent and child. First, unconditional love does not require anything in return. God does not need anything from us, which gives you the freedom to express ourselves openly to Him. If you need help, then ask for it loudly and specifically. Are you angry because our human limitations don't allow us to fully understand God's plan for us? Tell Him about it! It is okay to yell at Him and ask for guidance to better understand.

Second, unconditional love has no starting or ending time because it is measured by infinity — an immeasurable limit. God knows our future, our present, before we were in our mother's womb. He chose us before we chose Him. The parental love we give to our children is only a fraction of the amount of love God shares for us. It will always be awesome and beyond human expectation. There is no end, just eternal life.

Third, unconditional love is a condition-less state of the heart. It doesn't fluctuate with changing emotions. God will not hurt you or gossip about you. He will not belittle your accomplishments or judge you. He will stand beside you as your best friend so you never feel worthless or alone.

Lastly, unconditional love lives in our spirit and graces us with its presence each waking day. God gave us His son as the perfect role model for us to emulate. It shows us God's plan for each of us. It also allows us to love without our sense of sight or touch. The spirit moves freely to connect out hearts and minds so God can work through others.

I've been thinking about this definition of unconditional love all week since my presentation this past Monday. I recapped my blog writings in a 45-minute talk to about 80 St. Jude Church's Family Formation night parishioners. I was touched afterwards by complete strangers who took strength from my experience. I catch myself thinking my cancer and cancer treatment struggle happened to help others. I know it sounds crazy.

If we accept that God works through people, then is it possible that He is working through me to demonstrate that the pain and suffering we endure here is nothing compared to the suffering Jesus endured to give us salvation? This thought drives me to be positive about life. When I feel the aches and pains of life, I rub my finger along the crucifix of the rosary for a reminder of God's love that He sent His Son to die for our sins. Next time you feel the darkness overwhelming you and loneliness attempts to consume your every thought, look up at the cross and meditate on the faith-filled gift of eternal life.

Finally, our human mind, body, and spirit require the feeling of a physical connection — a well-timed hug, a kind word, or the sight of a dear friend. I cannot begin to name all the renewed friendships and newly formed friendships I experienced as a duck stuck in the ravine. To love a stranger, in turn, is to feel sad, frightened, concerned, angry, lost, and often helpless — and to do all this silently, for the most part, because you either didn't know what to say or were part of the medical staff and didn't want to break the professional barrier. Does it help you, my beloved ones, to know that I understand this? Believe me, I do recognize and deeply appreciate the incredibly high price you paid for loving me.

Every victory is yours as much as it is mine. Continue the fight and aim to be an unconditional friend. Together we can do amazing things!

CHAPTER EIGHTEEN

Good Employee?

Employers are recognizing that valuable employees are a rare commodity. Stephen R. Covey said, "Always treat your employees exactly as you want them to treat your best customers." It is often difficult to find and hire a good employee, though. Employers cannot afford to lose time, money, and results from a bad hiring choice. The cost of finding, interviewing, engaging, and training new employees is high. Employees require desks, computers, phones, and related equipment, in addition to the largest costs of being an employer — salaries, benefits, and taxes.

I went through this process when I was hired in August 2015 by a leading insurer with about 55,000 employees worldwide serving customers in global and local markets. They market themselves as a company whose employees give back to the communities where they live and work. They talk about their commitment to the employees who make all this happen.

I also like to believe employee loyalty begins with employer loyalty. Employees who believe that management is concerned about them as a whole person — not just an employee — are more productive, more satisfied, and more fulfilled. Satisfied employees mean satisfied customers, which leads to profitability.

I would like to think I was hired and rated high on my project contributions based on the following traits:

1 **Communicator:** I communicated well and expressed myself in a clear manner, in both writing and speaking.

2 **Self-Motivated:** I never hesitated to take responsibility. I worked beyond the call of duty to meet goals and to solve problems.

3 **Hard worker:** You would be challenged to find a single person who would question my dedication to my professionalism and commitment to completing each assignment with precision and perfection.

4 **Adaptable/decisive and effective learner:** I knew how to adjust myself to new environments and was willing to learn new things (quick learner) in the transition from the financial sector to the insurance sector.

5 **Team Player:** Bonded quickly and received recognition as an ideal team player from other senior managers in cooperating business units.

6 **Helping others:** Everyone needs a helping hand now and then. I did not hesitate to help others out. This established friendly relations with my co-workers and kept the office running smoothly, which the other employees appreciated.

7 **Honesty:** I was a good learner because of my ability to conduct self-reviews and my willingness to receive feedback (bad and good).

8 **Ethical:** Work rules are made to be followed. I followed the policies of the company and inspired others to do so.

9 **Polite:** Being friendly and approachable will never cause any harm.

10 **Disciplined and punctual:** Every boss likes a punctual, disciplined, and conscientious employee.

11 **Avoid gossip:** Everybody should always remember that we come to the office to work and to make a career. I respected the privacy of my co-workers and protected the confidential nature of office business and transactions.

I disclosed to my manager that a routine surgery had unfortunately turned out with devastating and shocking news. I had Stage IV Lymphoma that had metastasized into my spine and pelvis. Instead of the empathic and compassionate reaction I anticipated, I received instead a series of questions stopping just short of accusing me of knowing I had cancer as a pre-existing condition. I worked during my chemotherapy except for every other Thursday when I had my 10 1/2-hour infusion. I laced up my work shoes each and every day just to show my manager that cancer would not define who I was as an employee. Rarely did my manager ask about my condition, and when he did, it was definitely rehearsed as he could not sustain any lengthy conversation. I never asked for work to be reassigned and never missed a deadline. My manager asked on a few occasions if I would be better served by going on short-term disability. As I lost weight and facial hair, I don't think he liked my appearance, or perhaps it was jealousy because other executive managers would stop by my office and sincerely ask about my health.

On February 25, 2016, I was admitted to the hospital and placed in a medically-induced coma for nearly six weeks. On the life scale I became a very critical and fragile patient. My manager used this opportunity not to comfort my family but instead to contact my wife to voice his displeasure that he wasn't receiving weekly phone calls to update him on my progress. A year later she still recalls his rudeness on the call.

I had only worked in the new job for three months before the doctors discovered my cancer, so I didn't qualify for FMLA. Being employed less than a year also provided a loophole for the employer to "separate" from the employee at the 12-month mark from the start of the short-term disability date. Technically, my short-term disability date started on February 22, 2016.

On February 23, 2017, my manager suddenly didn't have the courage to look me in the eye, so to speak, and call me. Once again, he didn't bother to check on my well-being or wish me the best of luck in my recovery process. Keep in mind that I was not receiving any income or benefits from the company as I was paid through a third-party insurer for long-term disability. I know my manager well. He always has to be the hero. I'm sure he called a team meeting to say how hard he fought for me, but HR made their decision. So, almost on cue, a human resource person called me so that for the first time in my life I could hear the dreaded phrase, "You're fired!" When I asked if the manager knew already, she answered, "He is the one who made the decision."

What's the lesson learned? Well, cancer does keep on giving, but I keep on getting stronger by fighting with unbreakable faith. My former employer not only lost a great employee but the opportunity to be included in the most inspirational story told in the miracle of an ordinary guy. Too bad — customers really like those kinds of true stories!

MIRACLE OF AN ORDINARY GUY

CHAPTER NINETEEN

A Funny Story

I had been warned way before my hospital discharge date in August that the common cold would be difficult for my comprised body to adjust to. It turns out the doctors got this warning right. The cold symptoms started slowly about 10 days ago with a runny nose and a dry cough. This might sound silly, but my nose runs with any type of effort. It's part of my lungs being in respiratory distress, and it's become so common to my family and friends that no one really pays attention to it and simply passes a Kleenex. So, it was the cough that signaled that I was in trouble when I began to lose my standing tolerance.

I still have a few fears lingering from my illness — fever and hospitalization. Luckily, I never ran a fever during this cold period. Now, here's applying a lesson learned. I went to the doctor early to make sure pneumonia wasn't sneaking into my lungs. In years past, I probably would have never gone at all. But it turned out not to be pneumonia and was merely the nasty virus cycling through the country. I took a course of steroids to help my lungs handle the inflammation. It worked, and I am doing a lot better today. The cold did zap most of my energy including my writing time so I figured I would use the time to tell you a funny story.

In May of last year, I was still weening off the ventilator at the specialty hospital. The weening process is a very methodical process of x amount of time on the ventilator versus increasing amount on a trach collar, which is like an oxygen mask but instead of it going on your face it is applied over my trachea in my throat. It was at this point that I started to regain some of my humor as I realized that even though I was not in danger of dying overnight I was still in for a fight. I was able to speak then and developed a good relationship with the nursing and support staff.

Here's the joke set-up I learned from my friend Jeff decades ago and I worked it like a charm. The nurse came in and asked how I was doing. I gave her the quick update she needed to hear, then I ran my hand along my jaw line. I asked the nurse if she ever heard of a person with "dog jaw." She answered, "No." I rubbed my jaw line again and announced that I had it since childhood and feared it might have gotten a bit worse. The nurse looked at me with a questioning look. I asked her if she wanted to feel it with her hand so she knew what I was talking about. The nurse agreed and with some hesitation slowly placed her hand on my jaw near my chin. I said it was a bit low and she had to trace her finger up towards my ear. She had a deep and intense look on her face as she attempted to feel the dog jaw. As she approached my ear, I suddenly let out a series of dog barks "Roof! Roof! Roof!" The nurse must have jumped out of her shoes and 10 feet in the air! She laughed so much and I got playfully hit for scaring the life out of her.

The joke must have been a hit as the nurse and others started sending more "victims" into my room so they could see the patient with dog jaw.

Yes, I knew I was feeling better then as I am now.

MIRACLE OF AN ORDINARY GUY

CHAPTER TWENTY

The Last Cast

I am reminded this week of the fragility of life when a close friend's father passed away. I write, erase, and write again each week in an attempt to get my message just right with the hope the reader will take a small moment to digest the fact that the flame of life can be blown out instantly. My friend understood this from watching me struggle this past year, but more importantly, I had reminded him how lucky he was for all the moments he still had with his father living so close to him and for the relationship he continued to develop.

It is difficult at times to understand the fact that being human means living with a battle of emotions. The battle is a roller coaster ride of rainstorms and sunshine each with the ability to push us to the ends of darkness or the sparkling colors of Heaven. Whether it's a birth of your first child or the sudden loss of a loved one, the feelings go deep into our souls.

Life can be brutally, painfully hard. Where do we find the strength to continue? The answer is, in keeping our faith, because sometimes we are looking at what's going on in our hearts as the battle we face is faced within us. The battle to keep going, to get up, to put our feet on the floor every morning is the persistence of saying "I am going to keep trying." This is a battle no one ever sees because it is our inner self. It is the battle we face not to give in to doubt or despair, to worry, or to fear. Trust in God to take a baby step each day to move forward. God's grace is there for you.

Remember there are people here to support you. If you try to do it by yourself, you will get crushed. You need others more than ever — your mom, your wife, your son, and your brothers. Do you fear crying and leaning on each other. Together you are stronger than you will ever be alone.

I was reminded during my cancer battle that giving help is easier than asking for it. The giving part is easy because we can control it. Asking for help means we are vulnerable. We recognize our weakness. We show our soft target. The minute you open the soft spot of your heart, you gain strength. God works through people. God puts people in your life to give you the strength you need for these moments when times get tough.

I wrote the following poem when my brother passed away unexpectedly, and I want to share it with you:

> *You can shed tears that he is gone*
> *or you can smile because he has lived.*
> *You can close your eyes and pray that he will come back*
> *or you can open your eyes and see all he has left.*
> *Your heart can be empty because you can't see him*
> *or you can be full of love you shared.*
> *You can turn your back on tomorrow and live in the yesterday*
> *or you can be happy for tomorrow because of all he passed on to you.*

You can remember him and only that he is gone
  or you can cherish his memory and let it live on.
You can cry and close your mind, be empty, and turn
your back
  or you can do what he would want: Smile, Open your
  eyes, Live life, and Go on!

From a loving father I hear him yell to The Net Man, "Get the Frabill — it's time to fish!"

MIRACLE OF AN ORDINARY GUY

CHAPTER TWENTY-ONE

The Gift Box

I stared at the lone box centered under the artificial Christmas tree. The red paper patterned with white snowflakes seemed perfectly wrapped with its crisp triangular corners. The bow surrounding the box pushed up against the lower branches of the tree, but managed to stand out despite the lights capturing the hundreds of neon fireflies caught in time. The house slept with anticipation of Santa Claus bringing the family gifts sometime in the night. Yet, I remained awake fixated on the gift.

The day was long and my lungs hurt from a full day of effort. The more I leaned back in the recliner the clearer the gift became in my vision. I didn't remember seeing the gift earlier in the day and now I couldn't get it out of my sight. I closed my eyes and my mind raced with a gnawing pain of curiosity as to the contents of the box. I opened my eyes quickly expecting the box to be gone. It remained in the full view despite the LED bright lights and tinsel glitter. I slid slowly off the recliner onto the floor like sap running out of a maple tree. I battled the need for rest against the curiosity of seeing the address label and was hoping silently it was for me.

I closed my eyes a second time to muster the energy to roll into a crawling position — ready, set, and push. I opened my eyes and almost laughed out loud at my own amazement over how the little accomplishments such as being able to be on my all-fours brought me joy. I almost forgot a crucial element of this expedition. I reached up to turn the oxygen compressor dial to increase the level to 8 liters. I crawled the 12 feet to the tree before lowering myself to the ground on my right side. I straightened my right arm up and tucked my right ear against my bicep as a cushion to prop my head up. I didn't know how long I could last in this position so I quickly reached for the gift with my left hand and tipped it downwards to read the label.

I saw the perfectly placed bow centered on the square top but...no label. I did notice that the lid was wrapped separately from the main box. I rested. I took a second breath and pulled up on the lid corner and a glimmer of light appeared to shine from inside. I was running low on oxygen and knew I needed to crawl back to the chair. As I turned my head to check for fall hazards my arm pulled on the box. It seemed to tumble over in slow motion as the top came off, but it happened so quickly. I tried to catch the gift from crashing over while maintaining my own safety. The room filled with the bright light shooting from inside the box and hitting me in the face like a prize fighter getting caught by an unexpected left hook. My arm fell to the ground and my eyes shut.

After what seemed like a brief moment, I opened my eyes and sat up. I felt a warmness in my chest, and my vision was clear...

I am looking through the eyes of my boyhood on Christmas Eve 1970-something. I am in the basement of my Aunt Betty's house, and my cousins are gathered in each section of living space. An equal number of boys and girls: me, my brother Sonny, my cousins Joey, Anthony, and Richie versus my sisters Jenny and Sue, along with my cousins Debbie, Christie, and Tammy. The boys crowded around a pool table we weren't supposed to play on, and the girls, well, they waited to see what kind of victims they would become in our pranking ways. Oh, the girls' singing would have put an end to Snapchat before it became known to the world these days. I apologize to my sisters and cousins, but America's Got Talent has no room for us. In the real time of 40-plus years since these Christmas Eve parties, I can still reach out to each one of you and hear your voice.

We put so many miles on the rotary phone in that basement trying to call WLS radio station or singing the "Chick-a-boom" song that we never noticed Santa Claus walking down the stairs. Without a doubt, Santa brought magic to a bunch of young men and ladies when he arrived with a white bag full of toys for everyone! We need to put our investigative skills aside as to who disappeared every year for milk and smelled of cheap cologne and appreciate the goodwill of an adult willing to bring joy to children. I miss my cousins and aunts and uncles!

I blinked momentarily only to see the scene change to my first house as a boy and racing upstairs with my brother to grab our stockings. No matter the economic conditions for the year, Santa always packed the stockings to the brim. They were always a big deal. I didn't grow up with a close relationship with my brother, but these Christmas memories mean the most as I see them as though I lived them just yesterday. I miss my brother and sisters!

I'm sure I received great Christmas gifts, but I guess my mind isn't always clear in these dreams. I do know, however, that we always attended Christmas Eve Mass. I'm not the night owl of the family, but I managed to stay awake for the entire ceremony. The real reason — because perhaps this was the year church ran long enough for Santa to visit the tree before we arrived home. To this day, I still beat Santa home from mass, but he hit my house before I woke to deposit the toys moving like a thief in the night. Second, my mom always handmade and baked Swedish Tea Rings. The aroma of the cinnamon and brown sugar would radiate throughout the house and awaken the sleepiest of bodies. Hot out of the oven there could not be a better choice to hit your tummy after a morning full of gifts. Finally, I received a Nerf football each and every year. I don't remember any other gifts, but the footballs I do. Thanks, Mom!

I smiled and woke myself up. The room was dark and I saw only a haze full of glimmering light. I felt a comforting hand touching me and moved my head slowly and realized I was sitting in my recliner. I wanted to be scared because I last remember lying on the floor. But I heard an inner voice telling me strongly "Everything is okay."

I closed my eyes trying to return to my dream, but the tender hand squeezed to awaken me. I forced my eyes open, but no one was standing next to me. I looked again at the Christmas tree and found there was nothing beneath it.

I turned to my left to grab a drink of water and found the gift box resting on the small shelf. I stared at the box thinking this was crazy. I didn't remember carrying it over here. This time I could see a label. I flipped on my reading lamp and saw it printed with these words:

Infinity multiplied by infinity — take it to the depths of forever and you'll still only have a glimpse of how much I Love You. May each particle of light inside be a reminder of the number of times love touched your soul.

I turned the label over and saw it was signed: **GOD**.

I wish you all a very Merry Christmas and thank all of you for the support so many of you provide to my family and me. Each of you has helped to fill my box of love in your own unique way. I hope everyone finds a love-filled morning, each and every morning.

Life is a gift — unwrap it and live it to the fullest!

P.S. Although this chapter reads as a fiction, the idea was inspired by flashbacks I remembered while I was in my six-week coma. I remember a feeling of warmth and love each time I recalled the memory. I did my best to share a piece of happiness in hopes you will take a moment to recount your own childhood when time worked in your favor on the fun meter.

Note: For the movie romantics, the quote is partially borrowed from Meet Joe Black.

MIRACLE OF AN ORDINARY GUY

CHAPTER TWENTY-TWO

Summary Presentation

G od Bless You! It is a joy to sit here in front of you. I know what it's like to work all day, fight traffic, battle the kiddos at the dinner table, and rush out the door for family formation. Your day hasn't been too much different from mine, but I am hoping you can devote 45 minutes of your precious time to tonight's message on Jesus in the Eucharist.

I want to talk to you tonight about an experience that happened to me when I most needed God and how our Lord not only answered my desperate call but developed my listening skills to make God the heart of our home. This is an experience that is not about me, but I do have to share a bit of my battle in order to give confidence in my conclusions. Let me help you focus on the message with a parable titled "God will save me."

> There was a man who lived in a house next to a river.

> After a heavy storm, the water rose, and an announcement came over the radio urging locals to leave their houses before their homes were flooded.

> "Oh, no," said the man confidently to himself. "I am a religious man, I pray, God loves me, God will save me."

The water rose higher, and the man was forced to move into the second story of his house. A fellow in a row boat came along and called for the man to hurry and get into the boat.

"Oh, no, that won't be necessary," the man insisted. "I am a religious man, I pray, God loves me, God will save me."

Finally, the house was completely engulfed in water, and a helicopter swooped in to rescue the man, now perched on the roof.

Again he refused, saying, "I am a religious man, I pray, God loves me, God will save me."

Just then, a huge wave of water swept over the house, and the man drowned.

When he got to Heaven, he demanded an audience with God.

"Lord," he said, "I am a religious man, I pray. I thought you loved me. Why did this happen?'

"What do you mean?" the Heavenly Father asked. "I sent a radio announcement, a boat, and a helicopter, and you still wouldn't listen to me!"

Keep this parable in mind because we will come back to it.

My experience ties into Luke 17:11-19, which tells of Jesus healing 10 men with leprosy. It reads:

11 *Now on his way to Jerusalem, Jesus traveled along the border between Samaria and Galilee.*

12 *As he was going into a village, ten men who had leprosy[a] met him. They stood at a distance*

13 *and called out in a loud voice, "Jesus, Master, have pity on us!"*

14 *When he saw them, he said, "Go, show yourselves to the priests." And as they went, they were cleansed.*

15 *One of them, when he saw he was healed, came back, praising God in a loud voice.*

16 *He threw himself at Jesus' feet and thanked him — and he was a Samaritan.*

17 *Jesus asked, "Were not all ten cleansed? Where are the other nine?*

18 *Has no one returned to give praise to God except this foreigner?"*

19 *Then he said to him, "Rise and go; your faith has made you well."*

What we don't know is what happened to the other nine lepers. What we do know is that one came back to Jesus to glorify God and thank Him for this miraculous intervention in his life. It is at this point that Jesus makes a seemingly strange claim: "The one thankful leper is saved because of his faith — only the one." This means being healed of leprosy is not salvation. It was certainly a healing, but it was not itself salvation.

Giving thanks to God is necessary for our salvation.

1. A call to healing.

2. Relationships.

3. Thank you.

4. Get busy living.

POINT 1 — EVERY ENCOUNTER WITH JESUS IS A HEALING ENCOUNTER.

Let me share my experience with you.

In late August 2015, I had just completed my annual physical with my primary doctor with good news. My cholesterol levels were finally within the good range and my weight was down approximately 20 pounds since April. Before jumping off the table, I asked the doctor to take a quick look at a lump below my left armpit area.

I raised my left arm above my head as if I were reaching for a rung on a ladder. I used my right hand to grab the lump and explained that I had noticed it back in April but forgot to say anything about it. I didn't experience any pain from it and didn't think it grew at all but only became more noticeable due to the weight loss.

The doctor approached and grabbed the skin tissue, pushed it in circles and in and out. I reported no pain. We repeated the process of raising and lowering the arm followed by the prodding three or four times. He took his gloves off and started talking as he rinsed his hands. He diagnosed the lump as "lipoma." Lipoma is a benign tumor (not cancerous) most commonly found in adults 40–60 years of age. There is no known cause of a lipoma tumor, but I obviously didn't care for the description "fatty tissue." The doctor put me at ease by explaining that skinny people get lipoma tumors also — so HA!

I put my shirt on and was uttering the words "see you next year" when the doctor handed me the business card of a surgeon and said, "Go see this surgeon for a second opinion just to make sure."

Long story short, I had surgery in the first week of October that revealed the lump was not lipoma but Hodgkins Lymphoma, a finding confirmed later by The Cleveland Clinic. Here are the oddities of my numbers for you:

- † **The American Cancer Society estimates 1 in 2 males in the United States will develop an invasive site cancer.**

- † **1 in 417 males in the United States will develop Hodgkin Disease cancer.**

- † **The American Cancer Society classifies Hodgkin Lymphoma as RARE, accounting for only 0.5% of all new cancer cases in the US.**

- † **Hodgkin Lymphoma is further classified in four subgroups with a RARE 5.0% identified as nodular lymphocyte-predominant Hodgkin Lymphoma.**

The prognosis is good with a typical 90–100% remission rate with primary therapy.

So, here is the shocker. If the surgery wasn't enough, I started the battery of tests such as blood draws, bone marrow tests, CT and PET Scans. I went to see the oncologist to review the results and discovered my cancer was at Stage IV consuming my entire torso and penetrating my bones.

The treatment plan included 12 rounds of chemotherapy with a drug regimen called ABVD. To put this in perspective, the regimen consisted of the same chemical elements used in mustard gas used during World War II. It was toxic, but studies showed it to be effective.

The "B" chemical element in ABVD is Bleomycin. Bleomycin has rare serious side effects that only effect approximately 1 in 20 patients. The side effects include severe respiratory distress to the extent if the symptoms are not detected within two doses, the patient has a high potential for death to occur. I was administered nine doses before I was admitted to the hospital on February 25, 2016.

✝ I was admitted to a regular room for assessment, had trouble maintaining oxygen levels >85%, developed a fever of 106, and was submersed in ice baths and intubated.

✝ I then spent 6 weeks in the ICU as they attempted to diagnosis the cause of my life-threatening symptoms; during this time, I underwent surgery to insert an airway trach tube and a feeding tube.

✝ I was transferred to a specialty hospital for three-and-a-half months where I was weaned off the ventilator and began rehab for muscle atrophy and speech problems, including swallowing.

✝ I was transferred to an acute rehab hospital for five-and-a-half weeks where a lung-function test revealed the loss of nearly 80% of my lung capacity due to irreversible scarring (fibrosis).

✝ In August, some six months after I was scheduled for infusion #10, I finally came home in a wheelchair requiring 4L of oxygen with no movement and 8–10L of oxygen for standing, rolling the wheelchair, and eating. I require supplemental oxygen for everything you take a breath for.

To help you understand what happened next, I need to explain what my therapy sessions at the hospital were like. The scarring in my lungs restricts both of my lungs from expanding fully to allow me to get a deep breath, and the lung capacity is limited to holding 20% air volume. The best way I can explain how it feels is for you to imagine taking a belt and tying it around your chest and pulling it tight. Next, put on a swimmer's nose clamp to decrease the ability to take in air through your upper airway. Now, with the belt around your chest and the clamp on your nose, try to swallow some food, brush your teeth, or talk. Difficult? Well, you're not done yet: Now try to exercise!

That said, the pain I experienced in performing therapy was probably more mental than physical. I would get so worked up with anxiety on Friday night anticipating therapy to come the following Monday. Therapy session times were posted on the room door on the date of exercise. I looked at my posted therapy time with dread — waiting for the torture to begin. The knock came, and two therapists would enter with the intention of getting me simply to sit at the edge of the bed with my feet on the floor, knees bent with thighs parallel to the floor and back straight up at 90 degrees. The goal was to build core muscles and retrain my breathing pattern. But here's how I interpreted the therapy:

> My hands are bound behind my back with the back of my wrists touching and secured with a thick black nylon zip cord. I fight with what little muscle I have as the torturers attempt to lift me to the upright sitting position. I thrash about in their grip and attempt to plea that I'm not ready or that I need my music or even the truth that I feel like I can't breathe. They assure me my "numbers" are fine as they get me upright. Then, a rag is suddenly stretched across my mouth and I'm laid back in-to the bed as the water is poured on my face.

> Don't recognize my description? I'm being waterboarded like enemy prisoners of war. Water fills my mouth and nose at the same time, flooding my sinuses and esophagus causing a gag reflex to exhale the oxygen out of my lungs. The cloth around my face prevents any water from escaping. The constant flow of water prevents me from inhaling or exhaling any further oxygen without aspirating water. Thus, I am tortured with the fear and panic of drowning over and over without the reality of actually drowning.

By the time my therapy session ended, the therapist would straighten the sheets on my bed and put my blanket back on me and call it progress. I was exhausted from the torture and oftentimes left more discouraged than when they started.

Everyday this happened to me, and sometimes twice a day.

In one of my darkest moments in the hospital, I lay in bed alone and crying. I broke down and texted these words:

I'm in a bad mental state right now. Probably a good thing I have no mobility.

Followed by:

I don't want this life anymore. I'm alone, uncomfortable and things weren't sup-posed to be like this.

I prayed every night, always beginning with the Lord's Prayer and thanking him for the wonderful support of my family and friends who made time for me. But I began to question whether I truly knew how to pray. I broke my regular approach and talked to God as a friend:

Father, my heart is heavy. I feel like I have to carry the burden alone. My thoughts are occupied with an impending sense of doom. Words like "exhausted," "distraught," and "overwhelmed" seem to describe where I am. I am not sure how to let you carry my heavy load, so please show me how. Take it from me. Let me rest and be refreshed so my heart won't be so heavy in the morning.

On that Monday when I sent out those text messages offering my surrender I had just completed another therapy session. Oh, I wrestled those therapists so good (and raised such a ruckus in doing so) that the nurses' station had to call to ensure everyone was all right. I was worked up and angry. But therapy was over, and the therapists were working to straighten out my sheets, which were wound up tighter than a ball of yarn. They asked if they could stand me up for 30 seconds to fix the bed.

Remember, I was not able to stand at all at this point without a considerable amount of help. Thus, a large male had his hands under my arms in a bear hug to hold me up. I agreed to try so at least I would have a comfortable bed to return to. I pushed as hard as I could with my skeleton legs as I stood next to my bed. The therapist behind me wedged me against the bed, the wall behind me and a walker in front of me. He kept one hand on my chest and used the other hand to assist the other therapist with the sheets.

I felt a light breeze wash over my face ever so lightly and glanced toward the window, but it was still shut. My eyes were suddenly heavy. The tension in my body released as I pushed through the ground with my skeleton legs. I raised up to a normal standing position and closed my eyes as an absolute calmness presided over me. If I had been dying this experience would be absolute comfort. But, I wasn't dying. To the contrary, I experienced an energy light up my body and seem to connect to my mind. I opened my eyes with an inspirational thought: "You are doing it right." I would describe it as similar to the visualization techniques athletes use. I blinked and heard it again: "You are doing it right."

I then noticed there was no chaos in the room, only peace and calm. The main therapist stared at me from the other side of the bed.

Therapist: "Are you okay?"

Me: "Yes."

Therapist: "You look so calm. What changed?"

Me: "I can breathe!"

The second therapist put me back in bed and put the covers on me before they left the room. It took me only a split second to connect what happened.

God had answered my question!

POINT 2 — RELATIONSHIPS ARE RESTORED.

When Jesus performed the healing, He restored relationships in the life of each leper. Remember, the lepers were in terrible physical pain as their flesh was rotting away. Leprosy is a horrible disease. In the ancient world, the only treatment was absolute quarantine — completely cutting the leper off not only from strangers but from family and friends. People did not know how it was spreading and were justifiably terrified at the prospect of contracting it. The leper was completely isolated except from other lepers. These lepers knew about Jesus — the healer, the miracle worker, the teacher, the One who was not afraid of them! So, they approached: "Have mercy. Pity."

And Jesus did. The 10 were healed and could go home to their families. They could hug their parents, their spouses, their kids. They could touch them again — and be touched by them. They could go back to their jobs and care for their families. They did not have to beg anymore. They had their self-esteem back, their pride back, families back, and their lives back. Jesus did not just heal their bodies. He gave them back *everything*.

So, Jesus asked the 10th leper who came to thank Him where the other nine were. We assume they were running back to their families as fast as they could. They were so excited to have their life back that they probably didn't think about saying thanks.

I received the Sacrament of the Anointing of the Sick after I had been home from the hospital for about a month. I am still ill and live with a very comprised pulmonary condition called Acute Respiratory Distress Syndrome. The sacrament is spiritual in nature and designed to heal the wounds in our hearts and help us endure the suffering of sickness in order to achieve salvation. I am paraphrasing Thomas Aquinas when he said the sacrament's recipient might receive physical healing but only to the extent of achieving salvation.

My heart was lifted from the dungeons of self-pity with the energy of the Holy Spirit, the blessing of the sacrament, and this conversation with Father Michael:

Me: "Did this happen to me because I have sinned?"

Father: "Would you punish your own sons to the point of great pain and suffering?"

Me: "Of course not."

Father: "Do you love your sons more than God loves you?"

Me: "No."

Father: "Then why do you think God would punish you?"

POINT 3 — THANKSGIVING.

The third point directs us to give gratitude for life and healing to God. Jesus tells us directly that 10 lepers were healed but only one was saved. The one leper gave thanks to the Lord. In our daily lives, we gather as an assembly to give thanks to God for all the blessings we have received. The second part of Mass is the Liturgy of the Eucharist. It begins with an offering and preparation.

There are three major parts to the Eucharist:

1. The preparation of the gifts and the altar.

2. The Eucharistic prayer in which the bread and wine become the Body and Blood of Christ.

3. The Communion where the faithful receive the sacred elements for the salvation of their souls.

The Holy Eucharist is Jesus Christ. Is there any real difference between Jesus in Heaven and Jesus in the Eucharist? No. It is the same Jesus. The only difference is in *us*. We now on earth cannot see or touch Him with our senses. But that is not a limitation in Him; it is a limitation in us.

POINT 4 — GET BUSY LIVING.

Finally, Jesus tells the saved leper to stand and celebrate his salvation. The point: Live your life and share it.

I now understand some of life's greatest challenges are within us. Life is a battle — a constant fight just to hang in there and not allow "life" to beat you. Maybe you are consumed with illness and it takes every ounce of energy to get one foot out of bed to the floor. Maybe you have little kiddos and the fight is to get them into bed. Maybe you are fighting a job where you get no satisfaction and experience difficult times with coworkers. Maybe you are fighting relationships with family or friends. What is *your* fight?

Whatever your fight is remember this: The question is never how many times you get knocked down. It's the number of times you get back on your feet.

We cannot quit.

We must fight the good fight.

It's in the struggle of the fight that we get tougher.

Remember to take baby steps, one foot in front of the other… and breathe. Make every day count!

CONCLUSION — GET BUSY LIVING.

Grab a lighter or one of those "flickers" used to light a candle or the grill. Flick it.

See how quickly the flame appears and yet, in an instant, it is gone when you release the button. We take the fire for granted, except when the electricity goes out in a storm and we can't remember where we left the flicker. The flame isn't as easy to create now.

Our faith can be described as the flame. When it is easily available, it is convenient for us to be comforted by its warmth. What happens when an unexpected storm comes? Do you panic when you can't find the flame? Do you quickly point out how chaotic the world has become and begin looking for other shortcuts?

I treated my faith like the flicker in my hand. When I needed God in my life, I made a conscious effort to connect to Him and tried to listen only when it was convenient to my time line. My hospital stayed slammed the brakes on all distractors in life. Faith became the answer to my fear. The very real chance of death and the fear of God's judgment, the unknown, and not being loved surrounded me. It took that dark storm to release me from my earthly dependencies on "stuff" I thought was important to break down to the point that I actually talked to God and asked Him to relieve me of the darkness. It was only then that I saw the light was not controlled by me like the flame of a flicker. God showed me He was stronger than the darkness by revealing Himself.

The flame and the light are Jesus Christ.

MIRACLE OF AN ORDINARY GUY

CHAPTER TWENTY-THREE

Moment in Eternity

I find it difficult to find the words to explain how my illness and injury from the cancer treatment led me on a journey to understand suffering. I experience the two sides of human behavior at, of all places, mass. The positive side is in those people who, perhaps, have experienced suffering or treated someone close to them who has suffered. They do not shy away from me or hesitate to look me in the eyes to offer a kind word, gesture, or act.

The less positive side are those people who slide a bit further away when I sit down because of the oxygen tank I carry and the nasal cannula in my nose. It's not that they don't want to shake hands. It's that they don't want to look into my eyes and see the face of God reflecting back at them. They want to change me, but they can't, and it frustrates them. The only thing they can do is draw away in fear and sometimes feel anger and disappointment in God. Somehow the sick, the suffering, and the disabled remind them who we really are. It's part of human nature to push away sickness and suffering because it's everything we deny about ourselves. It's difficult for them to see God in people like me because they have never truly suffered.

So, where is God in the cries of starving children? Where is God in the father diagnosed with cancer? Where is God in the innocent victims of senseless acts of violence? The answer has always been hidden in plain sight with the question: Where is God in His Son who suffered and died on the cross? The resurrection is all the proof we need, to know that real power comes *only* through powerlessness. Death was defeated for eternity by one vulnerable act of powerlessness.

Suffering is the great problem of human life. We all have to suffer, as sorrows, sometimes small and sometimes greater, fall into our lives. We suffer from ill-health, from pains, headaches, anxiety, depression, from accidents, from enemies. We may have financial difficulties. Some suffer for weeks in their homes, some in hospitals, and others at work.

Why does God allow us to suffer? Simply because He is asking us to take a little share in His Passion. The Passion is not a statement of fact about suffering, a crucifixion, or a resurrection. The Passion is a story that must be told in its entirely so we can step into the experience, move around within it, and make it our own. Therefore, the story can be healing and liberating. I have struggled at times to understand the daily suffering I endured and how it relates to sin. I reflect and pray on John's story of Jesus' healing of a man born blind from physical blindness to sight and from spiritual blindness to spiritual insight.

This is a story about sin and how it sheds light on the sick, the disabled, and the suffering in the world. As Jesus and His disciples approached the man, the disciples question Jesus as to whose sin — the man's or his parents' — caused him to be born blind. Jesus answered, "Neither he nor his parents sinned. It is so the works of God can be visible through him." I like to think Jesus was telling the disciples and us that to look into the face of the sick, the suffering, and the disabled is to look into the face of God.

Suffering is not evil, for no one suffered more than the Son of God Himself, nor more than His Blessed Mother or the Saints. Every suffering comes from God. It may appear to come to us by chance or accident or from someone else, but in reality, every suffering comes to us from God. Nothing happens to us without His wish or permission. God suffered all the dreadful pains of His Passion for each one of us. How can we refuse to suffer a little for love of Him? This is the greatest lesson for us. It teaches us that we too must suffer.

So, how do we bear suffering? We must understand that what really makes suffering difficult to bear is our own impatience, our fight against it, our refusal to accept it. This irritation increases our sufferings a hundred-fold and robs us of our chance to do penance for our sins. The greater sufferings that fall within us from time to time become easy to bear if we accept them with calm and patience. God will give us abundant strength to bear our sufferings if only we ask Him. Through prayer, everything is possible. This is the secret of happiness.

I came across a great article discussing the difference between physical suffering and the physical disfigurement of the disabled. Deacon Errol Kissinger discussed an interview with an unidentified woman who cared for a disabled family member for more than 30 years. When she was asked how she made sense of suffering in the world, this was her response:

> If there was ever a pure, sinless human soul, it is the sick and the disabled. Why did they have to live a life like this? I said to myself, "I have to reconciled this if

I'm going to believe in a good God, in a kind God, and so I pondered and struggled with it and came out of it more or less this way."

There were two courses in college that meant more to me philosophically than any other two. One was astronomy because you get a vista of the cosmos and your perspective opens out to an absolute incredible degree. The other was anthropology where you get some idea of the development of the human being on this planet Earth. Both classes were exercises in perspective. So, I decided a human being's life is but a moment in eternity. To use a figure of speech about the caterpillar in the cocoon stage and the butterfly stage it is a very telling figure when you put it that together with our life on earth as a moment of eternity. Maybe this is the sick and disabled's moment in a cocoon. I have had a sense that I should somewhere, someday along the pathways of God meet them when they come into their own, and they come to me with rushing wings.

I can't help but feel that these people — people who are starving to death, oppressed, born crippled — will find true healing. Their time will come. In eternity, we are all but a moment in time. Many of us in our sickness and suffering have yet to come into our own, and for those who have, God calls us to nurture those who have not yet arrived.

If you are suffering, then pray to Our Lady of Sorrows for all your troubles. You need to ask her to help you. God gave her all the immense graces necessary to make her the perfect Mother of God, but He also gave her all the graces, the tenderness, and the love necessary to be our most perfect and loving Mother. No mother on Earth ever loved a child as Our Blessed Lady loves us.

Suffering endured calmly and patiently brings out all that is good in us. Those who have suffered are usually the most charming people!

MIRACLE OF AN ORDINARY GUY

CHAPTER TWENTY-FOUR

This Is Rex

The greatest fear dogs know is the fear that you will not come back when you go out the door without them. They are the only animals on Earth that love you more than they love themselves. I often wondered, as I listened to the late-night sounds of my ventilator humming, if my four-year-old chocolate Labrador Retriever named Rex missed me. A person can learn a lot from a dog, even a loopy one like mine.

Rex teaches me about living each day with unbridled exuberance and joy, about seizing the moment and following your heart. He teaches me to appreciate the simple things — a walk in the yard, the fresh smell of the lilac bush, or a nap in the middle of the day. He has a unique way of teaching me about optimism in the face of adversity by his sheer energy over nothingness. Rex reminds me about friendship and selflessness and, above all else, unwavering loyalty.

Let me tell you about Rex. He is trained well. My yard is approximately three-quarters of an acre with escape points at the far edge with a sidewalk used by dog walkers and joggers that runs parallel to a busy street. The longer edge borders my neighbor's yard, and the two on either side of my house are unfenced. I do not use an invisible fence. Rex just knows this is his boundary, and it works 90 percent of the time. The other

10 percent of the time can be blamed on his archenemies — the squirrel and the rabbit.

I like to think most squirrels and rabbits have nothing more on their mind than food. But the ones in my yard seem to be in cahoots with each other on their strategy to get Rex in trouble. The squirrel knows the exact distance he can stand from a tree and call on Rex to chase him. It is like watching a *Tom & Jerry* cartoon in which the dog is on a leash and Tom draws the line in the dirt so the dog races out of his dog house only to be yanked back by the leash. The rabbit on the other hand figured out — apparently from watching television — that people bet on dog races, and the rabbit they chase around the track always wins. The rabbit runs, Rex runs, and Rex comes back tired. This daily routine makes me wonder at times whether Rex were born not in a litter, but hatched from an egg of a dodo bird. I say this with all affection for my dog.

Rex shows some creativity also. He absolutely loves to be petted, especially his backside. He will do his best to show you his cute floppy ears and tilt his head in this magic way to get you hooked on his adorable features before quickly turning ever so slightly so that you are suddenly scratching his butt. Oh, and if this isn't enough, Rex will bury his head into the ground with his forearms flat on the floor and his butt clear up in the air as if to say, "This spot, Master. Scratch me here!"

He does have a final tactic if none of his other tricks work. He grabs his favorite bone made of hard white plastic and measuring about eight inches and rolls over on his back with the bone in his mouth. He flips the bone over to his side and slides on the carpet so it is centered on his back. He proceeds to roll over on the bone for minutes at a time while grunting to his satisfaction. Upon completion, he stands up and shakes. Every day he performs the show for me. He is so predictable. This is Rex with his favorite bone.

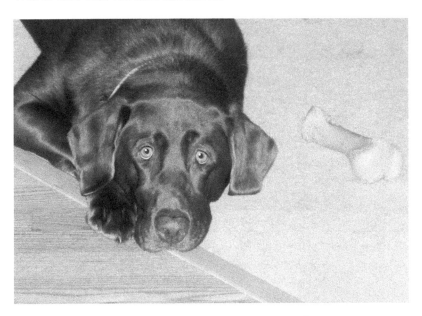

Rex is also an attention-seeker. I often put him in the kitchen with a child gate so I can get my therapy in without competing with Rex who wants his backside scratched. The problem is, Rex loves the female voice. He gets it in his head that they are actually here to see him. So, he figured out if he puts his head down like a charging bull he can move the gate, and, like magic, he appears in the therapy room waiting to be petted. Maybe as punishment, however, my boys can do anything in the world to Rex and he just lies there and tolerates it.

Here is Zach using Rex as his "body pillow":

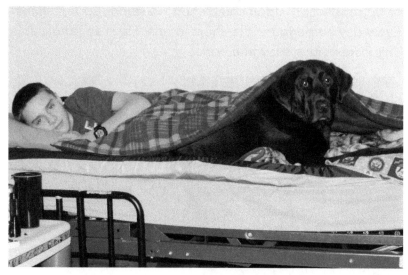

or Jacob using him as a "snuggle bunny":

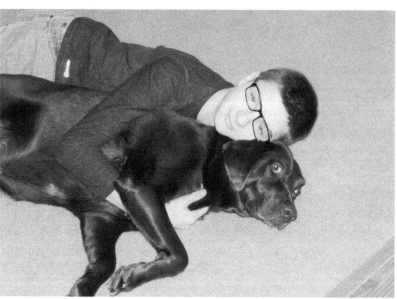

Lastly, Rex is not allowed on the furniture. He has been trained from the day of his hatching not to climb on couches and beds, but it doesn't stop him from trying to find the comforts of his family wherever he can. He has been known to rest his head on top of shoes, eat whole socks, or nap on sections of my blanket hanging on the floor. But, recently, Rex thinks he is my lap dog. As though he knows something I cannot see or feel, Rex becomes a master of creating an emotionally safe space just by being himself. It is as if something deep within my soul connects with his energy, his unwavering unconditional love and unrestrained joy. Rex makes me feel special and teaches me by example to enjoy simple pleasures and live totally in the moment. He teaches me there is only now and only who I am, who I am with, and what I am doing right now. Here is Rex, my 107-pound lap dog:

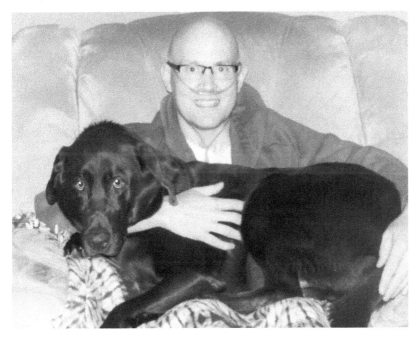

It's no wonder they call dogs man's best friend. Because dogs live in the present. Because dogs don't hold grudges. Because dogs let go of all their anger daily, hourly, and never let it fester. They absolve and forgive with each passing minute. Every turn of a corner is the opportunity for a clean slate. Every bounce of a ball brings joy and the promise of a fresh chase. Rex is faithful and loyal and true. He shares in my sorrows and rejoices with me in my triumphs, a better friend than I deserve.

Rex has refused to leave his master even when death and destruction lay all around me. Ah, noble dog, you are the furry mirror image in which I see my better self-reflected, a man as I can be, unstained by war or ambition, and unspoiled by a lack of character.

Yes, Rex, your master once again came home to you!

FOR MORE PICTURES AND MEMORIES, PLEASE VISIT:
WWW.MIKEALTENHOFF.COM

Acknowledgments

As I finish writing this book, I feel blessed in many ways for God's grace and His work performed through the actions of others.

I didn't want to use specific names and details of the people you have read about in these pages to not only protect their identities, but so the reader can easily personalize the story to their experience. I'm blessed to know the real people behind my stories who continue to inspire me to selflessly respond to my miracle. They remind me that Jesus is a family affair.

If this book challenges you to continue the fight by focusing your attention away from human distractions of stress and worry by remembering Hosea 11:8, "How can I abandon you? My love for you is too strong," then I have truly traveled the path God set sail for me.

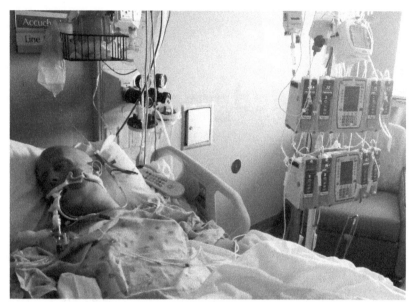

Mike on February 25, 2016

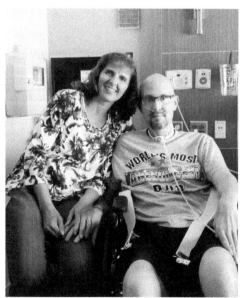

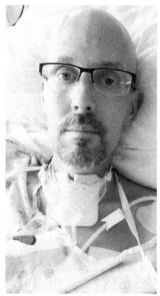

27th Wedding Anniversary

Mike on Ventilator at Specialty Hospital

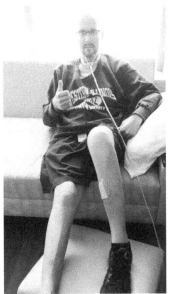

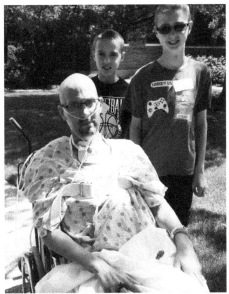

*Mike Graduating
Inpatient Therapy*

Mike's 1st Time Outside in 5 Months

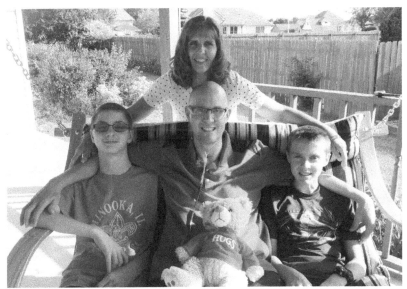

Focus on the Good in Your Life

CPSIA information can be obtained
at www.ICGtesting.com
Printed in the USA
BVHW01s0709090318
510098BV00025B/216/P